PROFILE PRODUCTIONS

CW00725179

Infant Feeding: the first year

Contributing Editors
Heather Cudby RGN RM HV Cert
Jill Leslie BSc SRD
Janet Thorne BSc Nutrition
John Wells BSc Nutrition

Illustrator
Justine Emmett

Editor
Jean Talbot MIHE

Publisher
Clive Whitfield

PROFILE PRODUCTIONS LIMITED   LONDON

Profile Productions Limited, 70 Elthorne Avenue, London W7 2JW
© Profile Productions Limited 1989

First published July 1989
Second impression February 1990

Infant Feeding: the first year

British Library Cataloguing in Publication Data

Infant Feeding.
  1. Babies feeding
  I. Cudby, Heather
  649.3

ISBN 1-871996-00-7

PROFILE PRODUCTIONS LIMITED

Infant Feeding: the first year

Contents

'Knowledge is of two kinds.

We know a subject ourselves or we know where

we can find information upon it'.

SAMUEL JOHNSON

Acknowledgement
Some of the basic material was first published in Feeding Children in the First Year, Edsall London 1979.

Department of Health
We have used DHSS for all reports, recommendations and events prior to the division of the Department in 1988. DOH is used for references subsequent to the division.

Editors note
At the time of going to press the Government's Principal Medical Officer had issued a warning about contracting salmonella from raw or undercooked eggs. It is important, therefore, that mothers are advised to cook eggs until the yolk is firm and not in the least runny.

Typography and distribution, Sylvia Meredith Services Ltd, 3 Elgin Road, Sutton, Surrey

Design and artwork, Sadlergraphics of Worthing

Printed by Stephens and George Ltd, Merthyr Tydfil

CHAPTER 1

Nutritional needs in pregnancy

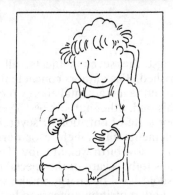

Feeding a baby starts in the womb. It therefore makes sense to consider the nutritional needs of pregnancy.

Pregnancy is a food consuming process. It involves the provision of nutrients for the growing fetus, the physical demands of labour, and the creation of a reserve store of energy for lactation.

In the past, much attention has been focused on achieving these aims by encouraging pregnant women to eat more food, though at the same time, advising against excess weight by the end of their pregnancies!

More recently, however, attention has been directed towards getting women 'fit for pregnancy'. They are advised to ensure that their diet is healthy and of high nutritional quality; that their body weight is within an accepted normal range for their height and build; and to abstain from smoking, drinking alcohol and taking unnecessary drugs. Doing all these things results in a greater likelihood of producing healthy full term infants of normal weights, and the avoidance of premature or low birth weight babies.

Energy needs in pregnancy

Calculations and dietary surveys which attempt to estimate the increased needs for energy during pregnancy are difficult to do, but it appears to be generally accepted that theoretically an extra 200 Calories a day throughout pregnancy is sufficient.[1] This takes into account the fact that most women, at least in the developed countries, tend to cut down on physical activity towards the end of their pregnancies.

This extra 200 Calories is not very much in terms of actual food, and normal day-to-day variations could be more, or less, than this. What women eat in practice is thought to be nearer their needs, with appetite their best guide.[2,3,4]

The problems of making calculations for increased energy needs are further compounded by the changes in energy metabolism which occur during pregnancy. Hormones produced by the feto-placental unit stimulate fat mobilisation, so that this can be used as an alternative fuel by the maternal tissues, leaving glucose available for the fetus.[5] This makes good biological sense, ensuring a buffer against possible deprivation in late pregnancy, when the demands of the growing fetus are dramatically increased.

The fact that women vary enormously in their energy needs during pregnancy has been well illustrated in a recent study by the Dunn Nutrition Unit at Cambridge.[6] The total energy cost of pregnancy varied from 104MJ (about 25,000 Calories) to 790MJ (about 190,000 Calories), a sevenfold range, amongst the seven subjects, all of whom were quite healthy and well nourished. The authors conclude that this high variability makes it impossible to prescribe incremental energy requirements for pregnant women in the UK.

This said, other authors [7,8,9,9A] emphasise that women who are definitely in a poor state of nutrition or severely underweight would benefit from caloric supplements either before or during pregnancy, in order to prevent them having a low birth weight baby. These authors emphasise the need for obstetricians to be aware of the special needs of their underweight patients.[10] The threshold level of energy intake which separates optimal fetal growth from fetal undernutrition appears to be around 1500 to 1800 Calories a day. Thus, although pregnant women do not now have to 'eat for two', they should at least eat enough for one.[11]

Weight gains in pregnancy

The most easily observed measurement of a woman's progress during pregnancy is her weight gain; but it is no longer sufficient to advise all pregnant women to achieve similar gains, or rates of weight gain, or to attempt to check rapid and large gains. More appropriately, weight gains in pregnancy are related to pre-pregnancy weights in order to achieve normal weight babies, although the relationship between these factors is still not entirely clear.[9]

Studies [12,13,14,15,16] suggest that mothers with a low pre-pregnancy weight require greater weight gains during pregnancy to achieve normal weight babies and adequate lactation. For women who are overweight before they become pregnant, the relationship is not so clear and possibly depends on the degree of overweight.[12]

It is generally agreed, however, that while large weight gains should be avoided, strict dieting before or during pregnancy could have a serious adverse effect on the fetus and is not recommended.[17,18] More appropriately, overweight women need to correct their body weights well before conceiving.

It used to be thought that overweight women who gained too much weight during pregnancy were more predisposed to pre-eclampsia, but this has now been shown not to be the case.[12,19] Similarly, there is not sufficient substantial evidence to suggest that excess weight gains during pregnancy lead to obesity in later life.[19,20] Hytten[19] advises that weight reduction during pregnancy is difficult enough, when the individual has to contend with a natural surge in appetite, and is of doubtful clinical value. There may be a case for intervention in the grossly obese woman, or if weight gain is abnormally excessive.

However, carrying excess body weight has its own disadvantages, whether pregnant or not. Extra strain is put on the heart, lungs, blood pressure and joints, and some seriously overweight people suffer severe psychological disadvantages.

Probably the best guide as to whether an individual is the right weight for her height is the Quetelet Index devised by Dr John Garrow.[20A] This is the ratio of the weight in kilograms divided by the square of the height in metres, i.e. Weight(kg) / Height(m^2). For example, a woman weighing 57 kg (9

6

stone), and 1.6 metres (5 ft 3 inches) tall, would have a Quetelet Index of 57 / 1.6², or 22.26.

Women whose Quetelet Index is less than 20 are defined as 'underweight', while those whose index is 30 or more may be termed 'severely obese'. Pre-pregnancy values which fall into either of these extremes may indicate that such women are at risk for complications of fertility and/or pregnancy. Further, Dr Pickard[20B] advises that normal weight women may need reassurance, as many of them regard themselves as 'too fat'.

Protein intake

The importance of a 'good protein intake during pregnancy' is firmly ingrained, but this has been based more on tradition than science.

Recent nutrition guidelines, such as the DHSS Committee on Medical Aspects Report,[20C] the National Advisory Committee on Nutrition Education,[20D] and the USA National Academy of Sciences Recommended Daily Allowances (RDA)[20E] have changed the emphasis regarding protein derived from animal sources in the diet. The trend is towards a decreased consumption of fat, sugar, alcohol and salt, and an increased intake of fruits, vegetables and whole grain cereals. Actual intake of protein is expected to remain much the same, i.e. around 10 to 15 per cent of the total Calories, but to come from a wider variety of food sources.

At present, official recommendations for pregnancy vary widely. The USA guidelines advise an increase of 70 per cent in protein intake, though the energy increase advised is only 15 per cent. The DHSS (1979) advises an increase of 26 per cent in protein and 12 per cent in energy.

Dietary surveys indicate what happens in practice. It would seem that many women eat considerably less protein during their pregnancies than the dietary guidelines advise,[21] but remain healthy and have normal pregnancies. Most women eat amounts which are consistent with the dietary guidelines for non-pregnant women.[9A] As with energy, there appear to be changes in aminoacid metabolism which are under hormonal, rather than dietary, control, and which ensure an adequate supply for the growing fetus.[5]

It is now generally accepted that protein requirements for pregnant women have been greatly exaggerated in the past.[9A,19,22] There seems to be no good reason for recommending intakes higher than those found in healthy non-pregnant women. The 1985 FAO/WHO 'safe' recommended level of protein intake for a woman weighing 60kg (132lb or 9st 6lb) who becomes pregnant is 51g daily (cited[9A]).

Extra protein is expensive, unnecessary and possibly harmful. Studies have shown that high protein supplements may result in more premature deliveries and low birth weight babies, due to intrauterine growth retardation. Other studies suggest that dietary protein is neither a cause of, nor a prophylactic measure against, the development of pre-eclampsia.[23]

In summary, there is little concern over protein intakes during pregnancy in the UK, except when overall food intake is very low. Those who might be at risk include some women of Asian origin who eat very little food, and women living in very poor conditions who probably eat too little of the right foods.[9A]

Vitamins, minerals and fibre

Although pregnant women in the past have, quite rightly, been advised to choose a diet of high nutritional quality in respect of vitamins and minerals, more emphasis recently has been given to some nutrients which, hitherto, have escaped the limelight. These include **zinc**, where a deficiency is now thought to be associated with low birth weight and certain birth defects.[24,25]

Calcium has always been considered important in pregnancy in terms of skeletal development, but more recently adequate calcium is thought to play an important part in preventing hypertension of pregnancy, which in turn may prevent eclampsia.[26,27]

Vitamin D status during pregnancy is of special importance in helping to prevent neonatal rickets, and attention needs to be paid either to the diet or to the climate.[28,29] Mothers who are likely to be of low vitamin D status before pregnancy need special attention.

Among this group are mothers of Asian origin, who may require special advice, as they are unlikely to receive sufficient vitamin D from sunlight in the UK. Vitamin D supplements are recommended for all Asian women of all sub-ethnic groups.[29A,29B] Some Asian women, especially those from Bangladesh, appear to have very little calcium in their diets.[29B] With this in mind, it would seem sensible to continue to fortify bread, one of their staple foods, with calcium. Some women from this group appear to have very low intakes of many nutrients, including energy,[29B,29C] and may need encouragement to eat more food during their pregnancies.

Vitamin B$_6$ (pyridoxin) appears to affect pregnancy outcome, though the relationship is not clear-cut.[30] There is no British RDA for pyridoxine in pregnancy or otherwise. The USA RDA for pregnancy is between 2 and 2.5mg (cited[31]), though it is doubtful whether most women's diets would supply this without supplements.

Pyridoxine requirements increase if the oral contraceptive pill is used, and it seems that this effect is carried over into pregnancy. Further, pyridoxine requirements are also directly related to protein intake. High dose supplements of pyridoxine, of the order of 50 to 100mg daily for a week or so, have been used successfully to treat nausea of pregnancy, and it may also be useful in the prevention and treatment of pre-eclampsia.[31] High doses of 500mg to 5g or more daily, and for long periods of time, such as a year or more, are dangerous, and toxic side-effects have been reported.[32,33]

Fibre is now a recognised essential component in the diet, and is especially important during pregnancy in order to prevent and treat constipation, which, although referred to as a 'minor complaint' by obstetricians, can be extremely troublesome for some individuals.

Special attention needs to be given to increasing the amounts of wholegrain breads, fibre-rich breakfast cereals and pasta, and fresh fruits and vegetables, as well as to drinking plenty of fluids. In many women, extra supplements of wheat bran have proved helpful.[34] However, care needs to be taken that the fibre content is not increased at the expense of the energy content of the diet.[4] Many high-fibre foods are filling, and a woman with a small appetite may risk not taking in sufficient Calories during her pregnancy.

Vegetarian diets

Provided that a wide variety of foods is eaten, a vegetarian diet can be just as healthy as one which includes meat, or even more so. Strict vegetarians (vegans) should pay special attention to their iron and zinc intakes, especially as absorption of these minerals may be hampered by the increased phytate of the diet. They also need to ensure supplementary vitamin B_{12}, especially during pregnancy.

Supplements during pregnancy

Iron: Iron supplements, with or without folate, with or without vitamin C, used to be given routinely to all women at almost the instant that the pregnancy was diagnosed. Now, such supplementation appears to be at the discretion of the GP. There is no 'official' policy.

Research indicates that there is no physiological basis for routine supplementation with iron for all pregnant women.[35,36] Some obstetricians therefore give iron supplements only when this is indicated by the blood picture, or if it is known that a mother is iron deficient before she becomes pregnant. It can therefore be seen that there is some value in screening women for iron deficiency at pre-conception clinics and correcting it at that time. Even then, prescribed supplements may be at a lower dose than has been previously used. This way, unpleasant side effects are avoided. The arguments against the widespread and 'indiscriminate' use of high dose iron supplements are based on the following considerations:

the absorption of iron during pregnancy is enhanced;

the increased blood volume of pregnancy should be taken into account when interpreting haemoglobin concentrations;

the absorption of zinc may be impaired and a red cell macrocytosis might be induced.

Studies of food intakes of women from Asian countries suggest that indications for iron supplementation are the same as for white British women.[29B]

The problem of iron supplementation is compounded by the fact that it is not always known whether women take the supplements regularly when they are prescribed. If iron supplements are given, these are best taken between meals, rather than with food, as they are better absorbed this way. Phosphates and tannates, which might be present in foods, can hinder absorption.[36] Constipation, diarrhoea and nausea are common side effects, and would deter the keenest mother-to-be. Such effects can be minimised by prescribing a smaller dose or a different iron salt, or by taking the iron supplement after, instead of between, meals.

Vegetable sources of supplementary iron offer a well tolerated source of iron with apparently no side effects. They are acceptable to vegetarians and vegans, who may especially need supplementation because they generally have lower blood haemoglobin levels. It should be noted that iron levels in these groups of women will be naturally lower, and this should be taken into account when doing blood assays.

Vitamin C, which enhances the absorption of iron, may be a more appropriate supplement.

Folic acid: Requirements for folic acid are increased during pregnancy, but at the same time, maternal metabolism of folic acid is also altered in order to meet these.[37]

It has been estimated that about half the pregnant women in the UK would become deficient, and thus run the risk of developing a megaloblastic anaemia, unless they took routine folic acid supplements.[38]

The value of such supplements has been open to debate because many women do not take them, and some studies suggest that the diet is adequate without them.[39] Nevertheless, many doctors recommend supplements of folic acid.

Prior to the introduction of routine folic acid supplements in the second and third trimesters of pregnancy, the incidence of megaloblastic anaemia of pregnancy was between 0.5 and 3.7 per cent.[40] Today it is not common in prosperous countries, and it has been suggested that in middle-class pregnant women, intake of the vitamin through diet is sufficient to meet the demands of pregnancy.

Of more interest have been recent suggestions that folic acid supplements, taken before conception, may be able to prevent the birth of a baby with a neural tube defect.[41]

Fluoride: It has been suggested that taking 1mg of sodium fluoride from the third to the ninth month of pregnancy, protects the teeth of the babies from decay.[42] However, some authorities feel that there is insufficient evidence of additional benefit.[45]

Some problems of pregnancy

Nausea and vomiting can affect many women in pregnancy and may be long lasting. If severe, some antiemetics can be prescribed; but small regular meals which contain a lot of starch, or are thickened by Instant Carobel (Cow & Gate), can also help. It has also been suggested that a diet which is high in protein (i.e. 70 to 100g protein daily) and low in carbohydrate, may make a mother more prone to sickness during pregnancy.[31] Further, if a mother has tried to reduce her weight before becoming pregnant by following a high protein, low carbohydrate diet, this too may make nausea more likely. Vitamin B_6 supplements and ginger may be useful.[31,31A] Hyperemesis gravidum is a serious condition which affects about two per cent of all pregnancies, and admission to hospital is necessary.[43]

Constipation is quite common during pregnancy, and as mentioned earlier, bran supplements and attention to diet may be necessary. Mild aperients may be given, but lubricants such as liquid paraffin should be avoided, as they interfere with the absorption of fat-soluble vitamins. Extra fluids can help.

Cramps may be due to circulatory changes and can be especially worrying at night. In cases where calcium intake is low, supplements in the form of calcium gluconate may be found effective.[44]

Heartburn can also be irksome at night, especially when lying down. Small, regular meals are best, with the avoidance of extra sweet foods. Some find that avoiding drinking tea or coffee immediately after or with a meal is also helpful. A glass of soda water or carbonated spring water may bring some relief. Sitting up in bed at night may be necessary.

References

1. Nutrition of the Pregnant Woman, 1973. Editorial. British Medical Journal, (5861) 255
2. Dobbing J, 1981. Maternal Nutrition in Pregnancy: Eating for Two? Editorial. Early Human Development, 5, 113–115
3. How Much Energy does a Pregnant Woman Need?, 1985. Nutrition Reviews, 43, (4), 110–111
4. Anderson A S and Lean M E J, 1986. Dietary Intakes in Pregnancy: a comparison between forty-nine Cambridgeshire women and current recommended intake. Human Nutrition: Applied Nutrition, 40A, (1), 40–48
5. Naismith D J, 1980. Maternal Nutrition and the Outcome of Pregnancy: a critical appraisal. Proceedings of the Nutrition Society, 39, (1), 1–4
6. Davies H L, Prentice A M, Coward W A et al, 1988. Individual Variation in the Energy Cost of Pregnancy. 2. Doubly-Labelled Water Method. Proceedings of the Nutrition Society, 47, (1), 45A (Abstract)
7. Viegas O A C, Scott P H, Cole T J et al, 1982. Dietary Protein-Energy Supplementation of Pregnant Asian Mothers at Sorrento, Birmingham. 1: Unselective during Second and Third Trimesters. British Medical Journal, 285, 589–592
8. Campbell-Brown M, 1983. Protein-Energy Supplements in Primigravid Women at Risk of Low Birth Weight. In: Nutrition in Pregnancy. Proceedings of the Tenth Study Group of the Royal College of Obstetricians and Gynaecologists, September 1982, ed. D M Campbell and M D G Gillmer. Pp 85–98. Publ: RCOG
9. Edwards L E, Alton I R, Barrada N I et al, 1979. Pregnancy and the Underweight Woman. American Journal of Obstetrics and Gynaecology, 135, 297
9A. Schofield C, Wheeler E and Stewart J, 1987. The Diets of Pregnant and Post-Pregnant Women in Different Social Groups in London and Edinburgh: Energy, Protein, Fat and Fibre. British Journal of Nutrition, 58, 369–381
10. Pregnancy in the Underweight Woman, 1980. Editorial. British Medical Journal, 1, 1154
11. Doyle W, Crawford M A, Laurance B M and Drury P, 1982. Dietary Survey during Pregnancy in a Low Socio-Economic Group. Human Nutrition: Applied Nutrition, 36A, 95–106
12. Borberg C et al, 1980. Obesity in Pregnancy: Dietary Advice and Neonatal Outcome. In: Topics in Paediatrics 2. Nutrition in Childhood Symposium. Ed. B Wharton. Publ. Pitman Medical Press, London
13. Luke B and Petrie R, 1980. Intrauterine Growth Correlation of Infant Birth Weight and Maternal Post Partum Weight. American Journal of Clinical Nutrition, 33, 3–9
14. Abrams B and Laros Jr R K, 1986. Prepregnancy Weight, Weight Gain and Birth Weight. American Journal of Obstetrics and Gynaecology, 154, (3), 503–509
15. Naismith D J and Ritchie C D, 1975. The Effect of Breast Feeding and Artificial Feeding on Body Weights of 42 Primiparous Women. Proceedings of the Nutrition Society, 34, (3), 116A. Abstract
16. Morgan J B, 1980. Nutrition During Pregnancy. British Nutrition Foundation Bulletin, No. 30, 5, (6), 300–308
17. Campbell D, 1983. Dietary Restriction in Obesity and its Effect on Neonatal Outcome. In: Nutrition in Pregnancy. Proceedings of the Tenth Study Group of the Royal College of Obstetricians and Gynaecologists, September 1982, ed. D M Campbell and M D G Gillmer. Publ. RCOG, pp 243–250
18. Campbell-Brown M, Johnstone F D and Kerr-Grieve J F, 1986. The Effect on Birth Weight of a High Protein, Low Carbohydrate Diet during Pregnancy. Proceedings of the Nutrition Society, 45, (3), 90A. Abstract

19. Hytten F E, 1979. Restriction of Weight Gain in Pregnancy: Is it Justified? Journal of Human Nutrition, **33**, 461
20. Beazley J M and Swinhoe J R, 1979. Body Weight in Parous Women: Is there any Alteration between Successive Pregnancies? Acta Obstetrica and Gynacologia Scandinavica, **58**, 45–47
20A. Garrow J S, 1981. Treat Obesity Seriously. A Clinical Manual. Publ. Churchill Livingstone, Edinburgh
20B. Pickard B, 1986. Feeding Children: In the Beginning – Nutrition and Pregnancy. Nutrition and Health, **4**, (3), 155–166
20C. DHSS, Committee on Medical Aspects of Food Policy, 1984. Report of the Panel on Diet in Relation to Cardiovascular Disease. Report on Health and Social Subjects No. 28, HMSO
20D. National Advisory Committee on Nutrition Education, 1983. Proposals for Nutritional Guidelines for Health Education in Britain. Health Education Council/British Nutrition Foundation
20E. NAS/NRC Recommended Dietary Allowances, 1979. National Academy of Science, National Research Council. Publ. Washington
21. Johnstone F D, 1983. Assessment of Dietary Intake and Dietary Advice in Pregnancy. In: Nutrition in Pregnancy. Proceedings of the Tenth Study Group of the Royal College of Obstetricians and Gynaecologists, September 1982, ed. D M Campbell and M D G Gillmer. Publ. RCOG, pp 9–18
22. Rush D, Stein Z and Susser M, 1980. Diet in Pregnancy: a Randomised Controlled Trial of Nutritional Supplements. Publ. Alan Liss, New York
23. Zlatnik F J and Burmeister L F, 1983. Dietary Protein and Pre-eclampsia. American Journal of Obstetrics and Gynaecology, **147**, (3), 345–346
24. Simmer K, Iles C, Slavin B et al, 1987. Maternal Nutrition and Intrauterine Growth Retardation. Human Nutrition: Clinical Nutrition, **41C**, 193–197
25. Flynn A, Martier S S, Millier R J et al, 1981. Zinc Status of Pregnant Alcoholic Women: a Determinant of Fetal Outcome. Lancet, (ii), (8220), 572–575
26. Belizan J M et al, 1983. Preliminary Evidence of the effect of Calcium Supplementation on Blood Pressure in Normal Pregnant Women. American Journal of Obstetrics and Gynaecology, **146**, (2), 175–180.
27. Repke J T, 1986. Pregnancy-Induced Hypertension: a Possible Role for Calcium. International Colloquium, L'Alimentation des Femmes Enceintes. Ed. J Rey and E Papiernik. Dept. Sante du CIDIL, Paris, 117–128
28. Delvin E E, Salle B L, Glorieux F H et al, 1986. Vitamin D Supplementation During Pregnancy: Effect on Neonatal Calcium Homeostasis. Journal of Pediatrics, **109**, (2), 328–333
29. Martinez M E, Salinas M, Navarro M P et al, 1986. The Effects of Season and Stage of Pregnancy on 25, Hydroxy Vitamin D Levels in Pregnant Women in Madrid. International Journal of Vitamin Research, **56**, 131–134
29A. DHSS, Present Day Practice in Infant Feeding: Third Report, 1988. Report on Health and Social Subjects No. 32. HMSO
29B. Wharton P A, Eaton P M and Wharton B A, 1984. Subethnic Variation in the Diets of Moslem, Sikh and Hindu Pregnant Women at Sorrento Maternity Hospital, Birmingham. British Journal of Nutrition, **52**, 469–476
29C. Eaton P M, Wharton P A and Wharton B A, 1984. Nutrient Intake of Pregnant Asian Women at Sorrento Maternity Hospital, Birmingham. British Journal of Nutrition, **52**, 457–468
30. Schuster K, Bailey L B and Mahan C S, 1984. Effect of Maternal Pyridoxine HCl Supplementation on the Vitamin B_6 Status of Mother and Infant and on Pregnancy Outcome. Journal of Nutrition, **114**, 977–988
31. Pickard B, 1982. Vitamin B_6 During Pregnancy. Nutrition and Health, **1**, (2), 78–84
31A. Personal Communication.
32. Alhadeff L, Gualtieri C and Lipton M, 1984. Toxic Effect of Water Soluble Vitamins. Nutrition Reviews, **42**, (2), 33–40

33. Sensory Neuropathy from Megadoses of Pyridoxine, 1984. Clinical Nutrition Cases. Nutrition Reviews, **42**, (2), 49–50
34. Anderson A S and Whichelow M, 1985. Constipation During Pregnancy: Dietary Fibre Intake and the Effect of Fibre Supplementation. Human Nutrition: Applied Nutrition, **39A**, (3), 202–207
35. Do All Pregnant Women Need Iron? 1978. Leading Article, British Medical Journal, **2**, 1317
36. Lind T, 1982. Iron Supplementation During Pregnancy. In: Nutrition in Pregnancy. Proceedings of the Tenth Study Group of the Royal College of Obstetricians and Gynaecologists, September, ed. D M Campbell and M D G Gillmer. Publ. RCOG, 1983, pp 181–191
37. Hytten F E and Leitch L, 1971. The Volume and Composition of the Blood. In: The Physiology of Human Pregnancy. 2nd Edition, 1–43. Publ. Blackwell, Oxford
38. British Nutrition Foundation, 1973. A Note on Pregnancy and Folic Acid. Bulletin No. 8, 18–20
39. McNulty H, McPartlin J M, Weir D G and Scott J M, 1987. Folate Catabolism in Normal Subjects. Human Nutrition: Applied Nutrition, **41A**, (5), 338–341
40. Rogozinski H, Ankers C, Lennon D et al, 1983. Folate Nutrition in Early Pregnancy. Human Nutrition: Applied Nutrition, **37A**, (5), 357–364
41. Laurance K M, James N, Miller N et al, 1981. Double-Blind Randomised Controlled Trial of Folate Treatment before Conception to Prevent Recurrence of Neural Tube Defects. British Medical Journal, **282**, 1509–1511
42. Glenn F B, Glenn W D and Duncan R C, 1983. Maternal Fluoride Safely Protects Offspring. Abstracted by Modern Medicine, **28**, (2), 80
43. Schulman P K, 1982. Hyperemesis Gravidum: An Approach to the Nutritional Aspects of Care. Journal of the American Dietetic Association, **80**, 577–578
44. Taylor K, 1980. How to Ease the Discomforts of a Normal Pregnancy. Modern Medicine, **25**, (10), 25–28
45. Health Education Council Policy Document on the Scientific Basis of Dental Health Education (1986)

CHAPTER 2

Outline of the physiology of feeding

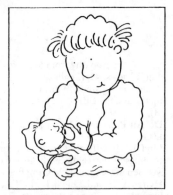

A baby extracts milk from the breast by rhythmic compression exerted by the jaw movements. Correct positioning of the baby onto the breast is important to prevent soreness of the nipples and to establish milk production.[1]

The capacity of the stomach is 30 to 90 ml at birth, 45 to 135 ml at one month, and 500 ml at two years. The glandular lining of the baby's stomach is relatively more developed than the muscular coats. The upper cardiac sphincter is weak, and regurgitated material can easily be expelled by vomiting. The pyloric sphincter is much stronger.

At birth the stomach contains amniotic fluid swallowed by the baby, plus a trace of hydrocholoric acid and digestive enzymes. From the moment of the first breath there is always air in the digestive tract.

As the food is passed through the small intestine by peristaltic movements, it is exposed to the action of various enzymes (Table 2.1). The transit time, or time it takes to pass through the whole digestive tract, is about 15 hours in a new born breast fed baby, increasing to as much as 28 hours in a baby fed on infant formula. This may explain why a breast fed baby in the early weeks often wakes more frequently than a bottle fed baby, and is less likely to sleep through the night.

The first evacuation of a new born baby is the meconium, which is smooth and dark green and contains mucus, bile, digestive juices and cast-off cells.

After a day or two of meconium, transitional stools appear, going from intense green black, through greeny brown, to the orange or greenish yellow of the breast fed baby's stools.[2,3] The frequency of defecation in breast fed babies can vary from four to six times a day in the early weeks, to as little as four to six times a week.

This variation does not occur in bottle fed babies, who are more likely to pass more formed stools, which may be green, from four to six times a day. Some milk formulas give rise to green stools with no ill effects other than the anxiety caused to the mother! Green stools can be an indication of underfeeding or overfeeding, but are not necessarily so.

Bulky stools may be an indication of overfeeding. Curds indicate poorly digested protein, and greasy stools indicate either an excess of fat or poor fat absorption.

Taste buds are present at birth, pre-term infants show a preference for sweet liquids,[4] and taste is well developed at two to three months, when changes in the flavour of milk will be noticed. But tastes considered unpleasant by adults, e.g. cod liver oil, are not necessarily rejected by babies. It is

TABLE 2.1   Outline plan of digestion and absorption in a baby's intestinal tract

Part of tract	Food digested	Activity	Enzyme involved
Mouth	Carbohydrate	Very little conversion of starch to maltose	Salivary amylase present at birth
Stomach	Carbohydrate	Conversion continues for a short time until inhibited by hydrochloric acid	Salivary amylase
	Fat	Small quantities of free fatty acids are liberated	Lingual lipase (secreted at the base of the tongue)
	Protein	Partial conversion to polypeptides	Pepsin
Small intestine	Carbohydrate	Starch → maltose + dextrins	Pancreatic amylase (fully active at approx 6 months)
		Dextrins → glucose	Sucrase - isomaltase
		Maltose → glucose	Maltase
		Sucrose → monosaccharides	Sucrase
		Lactose → monosaccharides	Lactase
	Fat	Conversion to fatty acids and monoglycerides	Pancreatic lipase (aided by bile) Bile salt stimulated lipase
	Protein	Conversion to polypeptides	Trypsin chymotrypsin
	Polypeptides	Conversion to amino acids	Carboxy- and amino-peptidases

thought that consciousness of textures plays a part in the acceptance or rejection of new foods, but just when this develops is not known.

Saliva is scanty during the first few weeks, and the salivary glands are not mature until the age of two years.

The extent to which a sense of smell is present in the newborn is not known, but babies have been known to turn towards their mothers' breast pads, rather than to clean pads or to other mothers' pads.[5] Smell appears to be closely associated with taste, and substances such as salt, acids and volatile oils must dissolve in the saliva and nasal secretions before they can be detected.

Teeth do not usually erupt until about five months, but the time scale varies greatly, depending on a number of factors including heredity. Teething should not be used as a developmental milestone, and delayed teething is not an indication of developmental retardation.

Babies whose teeth do not appear in the first year may have difficulties weaning onto hard and lumpy foods. Mothers should be advised to use caution with different textures until the teeth come through, but should offer them as soon as the baby can cope.

References

1. Marsh G N, 1985. Modern Obstetrics in General Practice. OUP
2. Barltrop D and Hillier R, 1974. Clinical evaluation of a new milk formula for infants. Practitioner, **212**, 129
3. Illingworth R S, 1968. The Normal Child. J and A Churchill, London
4. Tatzer E, Schubert M T, Timischl W and Simbruner G, 1985. Discrimination of taste and preference for sweet in premature babies. Early Human Development, **12**, 23–30
5. Macfarlen J A, 1975. Olfaction in the development of social preferences in the human neonate. In Parent-Infant Interaction. Ciba Foundation Symposium 33. Ciba Foundation, London

CHAPTER 3

An infant's nutritional needs

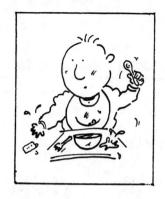

Energy

A major function of food is the provision of energy. The energy in food is supplied by protein, fat and carbohydrate at the following levels:

> 1g protein   = 17 kJ (4.0   kcal)
> 1g fat   = 37 kJ (9.0   kcal)
> 1g carbohydrate = 16 kJ (3.75 kcal)

Energy is required for the various processes occurring in the tissues, such as protein synthesis, the conduction of nerve impulses, building bones, and for muscular work and the maintenance of body temperature.

Theoretically, an infant's energy requirement may be estimated by the factorial method whereby the requirement for basal metabolism (energy expended while the body is completely at rest), physical activity and growth are individually determined and added together. However, in practice the growth and activity of infants vary considerably from one individual to another, and consequently it is usual to calculate energy requirements from the intake of breast milk or infant formula observed with healthy children who are growing normally.[1,2]

The recommended daily amounts of energy for infants and young children are given in Table 3.1. These recommended amounts are intended to be applied to groups or populations only, and the fact that an individual consumes more or less than the specified amount does not in itself indicate an over-adequate or inadequate intake, but it may justify further dietary or clinical investigation.

Protein

Protein is required for the maintenance and growth of body tissues. However, it will only be used for this purpose when the energy intake is adequate. When the intake of energy is insufficient, protein will be used as an energy source rather than for tissue synthesis.

Protein is continually lost from the body either as cells in the faeces or in the form of breakdown products, such as urea in urine. The protein required to replace these losses, the maintenance requirement, has been determined by experiment and amounts to 0.75g protein per kilogram per day (/kg/d).[2]

The protein required for growth is greatest during early infancy when the rate of growth is highest. The growth velocity reduces progressively through-

TABLE 3.1 Recommended daily amounts of energy and nutrients

	AGE (years)				
	0 to 0.5	**0.5 to 1**	**1 to 2**	**2 to 3**	**3 to 4**
Weight kg	6	9	11.5	13.5	16.5
lb	13	20	25	30	36
Energy kcal	kg× 108	kg× 100	1200	1400	1560
MJ	kg× 0.45	kg× 0.42	5.0	5.75	6.5
Protein g	kg× 2.7	kg× 2.5	30	35	39
Vitamin A activity µg retinol equiv.	450	450	300	300	300
Vitamin D µg cholecalciferol	7.5	7.5	10	10	10
Vitamin C mg	20	20	20	20	20
Nicotinic acid mg equiv.	5	5	7	8	9
Thiamin mg	0.3	0.3	0.5	0.6	0.6
Riboflavin mg	0.4	0.4	0.6	0.7	0.8
Calcium mg	600	600	600	600	600
Iron mg	6	6	7	7	8
Zinc mg	3.0	5.0	10.0	10.0	10.0

References: (Zinc)[25] (Other than zinc)[1]

out the first year of life, and is paralleled by a decline in the need for protein. Thus at 1–2, 5–6 and 9–12 months the protein required for growth is estimated to be 1.5, 0.6 and 0.4g/kg/d respectively.[2]

The recommended daily allowances for protein given in Table 3.1 adequately meet the estimated protein requirements, and also provide a safety margin to cover unforeseen circumstances.

An infant's protein intake will depend to a large extent on the type of milk consumed, since the proteins of human and cows' milk differ quantitatively and in type (Table 3.2).

A baby who consumes 150ml/kg/d of breast milk or infant formula will have a protein intake of between 1.8 and 2.9g/kg/d. When the same quantity of unmodified cows' milk is given, the protein intake is doubled to 5.2g/kg/d. Some of this extra protein is used for building tissues and leads to an accelerated growth pattern.[3]

However, not all the additional protein is used for this purpose, and large quantities of the absorbed amino acids are converted into urea, which is excreted by the kidneys.

The higher level of protein in cows' milk is a burden to a young baby's kidneys, and this is one reason why unmodified cows' milk should not be given to babies before the age of 6 months.

Unmodified cows' milk has a high content of casein, which forms a tough, rubbery curd in the infant's stomach. Breast milk, on the other hand, contains

TABLE 3.2: Main differences in nutrient levels
between cows' milk and mature breast milk
(Values per 100 ml)

		Cows' milk	Mature breast milk
Energy	kcal	63	70
Fat	g	3.7	4.2
Protein	g	3.2	1.3
casein : whey		80 : 20	40 : 60
Carbohydrate (lactose)	g	4.6	7.4
Sodium	mg	49	15
Potassium	mg	146	60
Chloride	mg	93	43
Calcium	mg	117	35
calcium : phosphorus		1.3 : 1	2.3 : 1
Vitamin A	μg	38	60
Vitamin D	μg	0.03	0.01
Vitamin E	μg	97	350
Vitamin C	mg	1.5	3.8

only a small amount of casein and forms a soft, flocculent curd.

Boiling cows' milk, and diluting with water, softens the curd and therefore reduces the risk of an intestinal obstruction. All formula milks are subjected to a heat process which modifies the protein so as to produce a fine, flocculent protein curd in the baby's stomach.

Taurine and cysteine are two amino acids which are found in foods of animal origin, including the milk of most species. A number of different biochemical roles have been identified for taurine, including conjugation with bile acids, retinal function and modulation of brain transmitters.

Adults can synthesise taurine from cysteine, but there is some doubt about the ability of newborn babies to carry out this biochemical conversion. Manufacturers of infant formulas now add taurine to their products to prevent the possibility of a deficiency.

Fat

Fat is a very important source of energy in an infant's diet, providing approximately 50 per cent of the energy in breast milk and infant formula. There is no specific quantitative requirement for fat in the diet. However, in addition to the provision of energy, some fat is essential for two reasons:

1. The fat soluble vitamins A, D, E and K require some fat in the diet for their intestinal absorption.

2. The body is unable to synthesise the fatty acids, linoleic and linolenic acids, and these must therefore be supplied in the diet. A deficiency of these essential fatty acids leads to growth retardation, the development of a type of eczema, hair loss and even death.[4] Breast milk and infant formulas contain an abundant supply of essential fatty acids. Thus a deficiency does not occur when either of these milks is fed, unless the absorption of fat is severely impaired, e.g. by cystic fibrosis.

The concentrations of fat in mature breast milk and in infant formulas are approximately the same. However, the fat content of breast milk varies throughout the day, and is at its lowest during the early hours of the morning. Also, within a feed the 'hind' milk is richer in fat than the 'fore' milk (see Chapter 4).

Babies do not absorb the fat of cows' milk as well as that of human milk. This is partly due to the higher content of long chain saturated fatty acids in cows' milk, and the low activity of pancreatic lipase and small amounts of bile salts in the intestine of newborn babies. Research with low birth weight infants has shown that short chain fatty acids are better absorbed than long chain fatty acids, and unsaturated fatty acids are better absorbed than saturated fatty acids of the same chain length.[5,6]

Thus during the manufacture of infant formulas based on cows' milk, the milk fat is replaced by a mixture of vegetable oils or a blend of vegetable and animal fats, to ensure good fat absorption. Excessive amounts of polyunsaturated fatty acids in infant formula are undesirable, since these result in abnormally high levels of polyunsaturated fats in the infant's adipose tissues.[7]

The significance of this effect in relation to short or long term health is unknown. As a precaution, however, the DOH recommends a maximum level of 20 per cent linoleic acid in the fat blend of infant formulas.[8]

Carbohydrate

Human and cows' milk contain on average 7.4g and 4.8g carbohydrate respectively per 100ml. This is in the form of lactose, a disaccharide, which is hydrolysed in the intestine to its constituent monosaccharides, glucose and galactose, before absorption. Lactose is not generally considered to be an essential nutrient because galactose, which is necessary for the formation of certain compounds in the brain, can be made from glucose in the liver.

Before the introduction of modern infant formulas, cows' milk was adapted for infant feeding by diluting with water and adjusting the carbohydrate level to that of human milk with sugar (sucrose). The use of sugar in infant feeds is now generally considered to be undesirable, since it is thought to encourage a taste for sweet foods.[29]

Lactose is the nutritionally preferred carbohydrate source for infants, for the following reasons:

1. It has a less sweet taste than sucrose.

2. Studies indicate that lactose encourages an intestinal flora rich in lactobacilli.[9] This is thought to help prevent infection (gastroenteritis).

3. Research with animals shows that relative to other carbohydrates, lactose may increase the absorption of calcium and magnesium in the intestine.[8]

Maltodextrin and glucose syrups are two types of carbohydrate which are prepared industrially by the partial hydrolysis (breakdown) of starch. These substances are ingredients of some infant formulas, e.g. Farleys' Ostermilk 2 and Formula S, and they are well tolerated by infants, even those born prematurely.

The digestion of starch may present a problem to young infants aged less than 6 months, who have low levels of the digestive enzyme amylase. For this reason, caution should be exercised in the use of starch either as a supplement or as an ingredient of infant formulas.[10,11]

Minerals

Some twenty or so mineral elements are essential for health, but only eight will be considered here since these are particularly relevant to infant nutrition. The mineral contents of human and cows' milk are shown in Table 3.2.

Calcium and phosphorus are the main building elements of bone. Cows' milk contains approximately four times as much calcium as human milk, and six times as much phosphorus. However, the calcium and phosphorus in human milk are more efficiently absorbed, and a higher proportion of the absorbed phosphorus is retained by the body.

As mentioned previously, cows' milk fat is not well absorbed by young babies, and most infant formulas available during the 1970's contained only this form of fat. Babies fed with these older style formulas occasionally suffered neonatal tetany (uncontrolled muscular spasms) caused by an imbalance in the amounts of absorbed calcium and phosphorus. One possible explanation is that undigested fat passing through the intestine combines with some of the dietary calcium to form insoluble substances (calcium soaps) which are unavailable to the body. The undigested fat does not interfere with the absorption of phosphorus, but since young infants have a limited ability to excrete phosphorus in their urine, a high level of phosphorus and a low level of calcium develop in the blood.

The recommended daily allowance of calcium for bottle fed infants in the first year of life is 600mg. There is no recommended allowance for phosphorus, but an intake providing a calcium:phosphorus ratio of 2.3:1, as found in breast milk, is considered optimal.[8]

Sodium and potassium are present in milk in amounts sufficient to meet the body's requirements. In the body, sodium is found mainly in the blood plasma, lymph and in the fluid present in the intercellular spaces, while potassium occurs predominantly inside the cells. Sodium and potassium are intimately concerned with the regulation of body fluids.

Cows' milk contains approximately four times as much sodium as human milk, and in the manufacture of infant formula an acceptably low level is achieved by the dilution effect when other ingredients are added to the formulation, e.g. lactose, or by electrodialysis of whey protein.

The older types of formulas available in the 1970's contained levels of sodium similar to cows' milk. Under normal circumstances an infant was able to excrete the excess sodium in the urine, but when insufficient water was given, either when making up the milk feed (over-concentration) or as drinks between feeds, hyperosmolar dehydration occasionally occurred. Conditions where there are excessive fluid losses, such as colds or diarrhoea, exacerbate the situation.

Recognising the dangers of excessive sodium in infant diets, a DHSS report[12] recommended that milks for babies should have a sodium concentration similar to that of breast milk, and that mothers should not add salt to solid foods fed to infants. All present-day infant formulas and manufactured weaning foods comply with the principle of this recommendation.

Iron is not present in significant amounts in either human or cows' milk, and this is one reason for introducing solid foods at about 4 months, as by then much of the baby's iron store, present at birth, will be depleted. Full term infants receive sufficient iron from their mothers to last 3–4 months. However, since a large proportion of this iron is passed to the fetus during the last few weeks of gestation, premature infants are usually born with low iron reserves, and they require iron supplements to achieve an intake of 2.0–2.5mg/kg/d (maximum 15mg Fe per day) from not later than 8 weeks of age.[13]

Iron is added to all infant formulas, and the small amount present in breast milk is very efficiently absorbed. Thus young infants normally receive sufficient iron. With older infants and toddlers, however, the weaning diet can often be deficient in iron, and iron deficiency anaemia is common, especially in those from disadvantaged backgrounds.[14,15] This nutritional deficiency is serious because it not only causes low haemoglobin levels, but more importantly it adversely affects weight gain and psychomotor development of the child.[16]

Zinc is present at similar levels in human and cows' milk. However, 90 per cent of the zinc in cows' milk is bound as a complex to proteins which are high in molecular weight, while in human milk, zinc is bound to low molecular weight proteins. It is for this reason that the zinc in human milk is more easily absorbed. Zinc is necessary for the normal activity of a wide range of enzymes, and a deficiency may result in growth retardation, skin rashes, anorexia, poor wound healing and other effects.[4]

Little information is available on the zinc requirements of infants, but the amounts supplied by human and cows' milks $(200-600\mu g/100ml)$ appear to be sufficient.[8]

Copper is stored mainly in the liver, and plays an important role in several enzyme systems. For example, a source of dietary copper is necessary for the proper utilisation of iron within the body. The clinical features of copper deficiency in infants include psychomotor retardation, hypotonia, pallor, hypopigmentation of skin and hair, and bone disease. Copper deficiency is unknown in exclusively breast fed infants, and most infant formulas freely available since 1983 contain adequate amounts.[17] Low birth weight infants are at greater risk of becoming deficient in copper, because they have lower stores at birth.[18]

The DHSS has proposed a tentative guideline of $10-60\mu g/100ml$ for copper in infant formulas.[8] However, this proposal has been criticised by Shaw[18], since manufacturers did not consider it necessary to add copper to infant formulas, and one low birth weight formula in particular was considered to contain an inadequate amount.

Fluoride accumulates in the hard tissues of the body, the bones and teeth, and this occurs more rapidly in growing children than in adults. Breast milk contains very small amounts of fluoride, and this appears to be unaffected by water fluoridation.[8]

Epidemiological studies have shown that the consumption of water containing 1ppm fluoride reduces the incidence of dental caries by up to 70 per cent.[19] Although powdered baby milk reconstituted with such water would provide an infant with approximately 10 times as much fluoride as is present in breast milk, there is no evidence that this is in any way harmful.

In areas where the fluoride content of tap water is less than 0.3ppm, daily supplements of fluoride are recommended throughout the period of tooth development from shortly after birth until adolescence, as follows:[19]

0–2 years	0.25mg F	(0.55mg sodium fluoride)
2–4 years	0.5 mg F	(1.1 mg sodium fluoride)
4–12 years	1.0 mg F	(2.2 mg sodium fluoride)

Parents should be advised to store fluoride drops and tablets out of reach of children and to avoid over-dosage, which may cause mottling of the teeth.

Vitamins

Vitamins are organic compounds which are required in trace amounts in the diet. The vitamins needed by man are broadly classified into the fat soluble vitamins, which are mainly associated with fatty foods, and the water soluble vitamins. The fat soluble vitamins consist of vitamins A, D, E and K and the water soluble vitamins of C and the B complex. The latter group comprises thiamin (B_1), riboflavin (B_2), nicotinic acid (niacin), vitamin B_6 (pyrodixine), folic acid, vitamin B_{12}, biotin and pantothenic acid.

Water soluble vitamins are not stored in the body, and any excess is largely excreted in the urine. One the other hand, an excessive intake of fat soluble vitamins is stored and in some instances can cause poisoning. The stores of fat soluble vitamins in the body delay the appearance of deficiency signs for a considerable time after the intake has become inadequate.

Normal full term infants who are breast fed or receiving infant formula obtain sufficient vitamins, and therefore a deficiency is rare in British infants. However, the infants who are most at risk are those who are breast fed by a mother who has a poor vitamin status.[21] Asian babies and premature babies are also more likely to suffer from vitamin deficiencies.

As a safeguard, the DOH makes available supplementary vitamins for infants and young children as part of the Welfare Food Scheme. The recommended daily dose of 5 drops contains the following levels of vitamins:

Vitamin A	$200\mu g$
Vitamin C	20mg
Vitamin D	$7\mu g$

The DHSS recommends that vitamin supplements are given to infants and young children from the age of 6 months until at least 2 years, and preferably 5 years. Earlier introduction of vitamin supplements is only justified if there are any doubts about the infant's intake at this time.

Fat soluble vitamins

Vitamin A has the chemical name **retinol** and is found only in animal foods such as milk, eggs, liver and fish liver oils. The orange and yellow plant colours called **carotenes**, which occur widely in green and red vegetables, have vitamin A activity since they can be converted in the body to retinol. The most important carotene, beta (β-) carotene, has one-sixth the vitamin activity of retinol. The vitamin activity of a diet which normally contains both retinol and carotenes is expressed in **retinol equivalents**. This is calculated by adding one-sixth of the level of β-carotene to the retinol content.

Vitamin A is essential for vision in dim light, and for maintaining the skin and the lining of secretory ducts in a healthy condition. A deficiency causes night blindness or total blindness and dry rough skin.

Acute poisoning may result from a single large dose of about $100,000\mu g$ retinol and causes vomiting. Recovery is spontaneous when the large dosage is discontinued. Chronic poisoning can occur within a few weeks when infants are given doses of approximately $20,000\mu g$ retinol per day. Symptoms include coarse and sparse hair, dry and rough skin and cracked lips.

Infants breast fed by well nourished mothers have an adequate intake of vitamin A. All approved artificial milks contain added vitamin A, to ensure a satisfactory intake when the quantity of milk consumed is sufficient to meet the requirements for energy.

Additional vitamin A, in the form of DOH vitamin drops or cod liver oil, is usually recommended as a safeguard against deficiency,[20,21] and is especially necessary for those infants who are poor feeders or those who have malabsorption problems.

Vitamin D is found at levels of dietary significance in relatively few foods. These include fortified baby cereals, eggs, butter, margarine, fatty fish and cod liver oil. Vitamin D is also obtained when the skin is exposed to the ultraviolet radiation of sunlight.

Vitamin D is necessary for promoting the intestinal absorption of calcium and for regulating the interchange of calcium between blood and bone.

A deficiency in infants causes the disease of rickets. The rachitic infant sleeps poorly, is restless and develops bowing of the arms and legs or knock knees. Historically, rickets was more frequently seen in children of industrial cities, where a lack of dietary vitamin D was not made good by exposure to sunlight.

Although the cause of rickets is now known, the disease still occurs occasionally. In previous years, the children of Asian immigrants appeared to have been affected more than others. However, there is now evidence that rickets in this group has declined following the greater use of vitamin D supplements.[22,23]

Unfortified cows' milk contains negligible amounts of vitamin D and all infant formulas are fortified to a level of approximately $1\mu g/100ml$. The level of vitamin D in breast milk appears to be below that required to prevent the development of rickets. However, the majority of breast fed infants do not suffer from rickets. The reason for this is unclear, but the alleged presence of the water soluble form, vitamin D sulphate, has now been discounted as a source of vitamin D activity.[24]

An excessive intake of vitamin D is dangerous, since it causes more calcium to be absorbed than can be excreted, and the level of calcium in the blood becomes abnormally high (hypercalcaemia). The hypercalcaemic baby is irritable and suffers with anorexia, constipation, vomiting and failure to thrive. If left untreated, calcium deposits in the kidneys and eventually renal failure will occur. Infants with vitamin D overload should be fed a low calcium diet to which no vitamin D has been added.

Vitamin E is present at high levels in vegetable oils, cereal products and eggs. Animal fats, fruits and vegetables contain small amounts. Vitamin E is necessary for normal fertility in rats, but in man this function has not been demonstrated.

A deficiency of vitamin E in man is very rare, and thus the effects have not been clearly defined. The level of vitamin E in the blood tends to be low at birth, particularly in low birth weight infants. The need for vitamin E is increased by a diet rich in polyunsaturated fatty acids, and a deficiency in these circumstances results in the development of a haemolytic type of anaemia. Infant formula manufacturers ensure an adequate level of vitamin E in their products by maintaining a minimum ratio of vitamin E:polyunsaturated fatty acids of 0.4:1.02.

Excessive intakes of vitamin E do not appear to be toxic.

Vitamin K is obtained mainly from intestinal bacterial synthesis. It occurs in a wide range of vegetable foods such as spinach, cauliflower, peas and cereals. A deficiency is therefore unlikely in adults who consume a mixed diet.

Vitamin K is essential for normal clotting of the blood, and a deficiency causes bleeding from the gums, nose or intestine.

Breast milk is a poor source of vitamin K, and during the first few days of life, when the gut is sterile, the intake may be inadequate. In some hospitals it is routine practice to give the newborn a prophylactic dose of vitamin K to minimise the incidence of haemorrhagic disease.

An excess dose of some forms of vitamin K preparations may cause the destruction of red blood cells (haemolysis) and anaemia.

Water soluble vitamins

Vitamin C (ascorbic acid) occurs mainly in fruits and vegetables. Rich sources include: citrus fruits, blackcurrants, strawberries, green leafy vegetables, cauliflower, tomatoes and potatoes. In the average adult diet, potatoes supply one-quarter of our vitamin C intake.

Vitamin C is one of the less stable vitamins, and is readily lost from fresh foods during storage or when food is cooked. For this reason, and because it occurs mainly in seasonal foods, the British diet may become deficient in vitamin C at certain times of the year.

Vitamin C is necessary for the maintenance of healthy connective tissue and increases the efficiency of iron absorption in the gut. A deficiency causes the disease scurvy, which is characterised in infants by tenderness and swelling of the legs, haemorrhage at the sites of recently erupted teeth, fretfulness, pallor and loss of appetite.

The recommended intake of vitamin C for a baby during the first year is 20mg per day. This quantity is supplied by approximately 500ml of human breast milk. It can also be obtained from all approved formula milks which contain added vitamin C (Table 7.1). Ordinary cows' milk is a poor source of this vitamin, so when the baby ceases to be wholly breast fed or wholly bottle fed, weaning foods containing vitamin C must be given daily. Ideally, fresh food sources are best, but unfortunately vitamin C is so easily lost in storage and cooking that it is probably wise to recommend vitamin drops, fortified fruit juices or fruit desserts, where the presence of adequate quantities of vitamin C are assured.

An excessive intake of vitamin C is rapidly excreted in the urine, and is harmless except when given in very large amounts.

Vitamin B complex Vitamins belonging to this group function as co-factors in various enzyme systems of the body. Certain foods such as cereals and meats are important sources of several of the B vitamins, and therefore an inadequate diet often causes more than one deficiency disease.

(i) **Thiamin (vitamin B₁)** occurs in a wide variety of foods. Good sources include milk, offal, meats, fortified baby cereals, whole grain products, pulses and eggs.

Thiamin is necessary for the release of energy from carbohydrate. Its requirements therefore are related directly to the carbohydrate intake, and indirectly to the amount of energy in the diet. The deficiency disease beriberi has been a major problem in communities that use white polished rice as a staple food. Infants fed at the breast of thiamin deficient mothers also suffer with beriberi because the milk has an abnormally low thiamin content. However, due to preventive measures introduced since World War II, the occurrence of beriberi worldwide has diminished significantly.

(ii) **Riboflavin (vitamin B₂)** The best sources include liver, milk, eggs and green vegetables. Milk is the most important source of riboflavin and, theoretically, supplies one-third of the total intake in the average British diet. However, riboflavin is destroyed by exposure to light, and it is therefore important to remove milk bottles from the doorstep as soon as possible after they are delivered. Failure to do so, combined with the length of time that milk may sit on a delivery float, makes it difficult to assess the actual intake from this source.

Riboflavin is necessary for the utilisation of the energy in our food. A deficiency causes the skin to become red and scaly in the areas where the sebaceous glands are prominent, nasolabial folds, external ears, eyelids and genitalia. Painful fissures develop at the angles of the mouth (angular stomatitis) and lips (cheilosis), and these may become infected with *Candida albicans*. Death due to riboflavin deficiency is unknown.

The requirements for riboflavin are met from a normal intake of either breast milk or infant formula.

(iii) **Nicotinic acid (niacin)** is another B vitamin which is involved with the utilisation of food energy. The body can make nicotinic acid from the amino acid tryptophan, which is present in food proteins. However, 60mg of tryptophan are required to make 1mg of nicotinic acid. The nicotinic acid content of foods is therefore expressed in nicotinic acid equivalents, and is calculated by adding one-sixtieth of the tryptophan content to the nicotinic acid content.

Meat, fish, wholemeal cereals and pulses are good sources of nicotinic acid, but in maize and other cereals a large proportion of the vitamin occurs in a bound unabsorbable form.

Nicotinic acid deficiency causes pellagra, a disease characterised by a dark and scaly skin, especially where it is exposed to light, a painful and swollen tongue, gastritis and malabsorption.

The recommended daily intake of nicotinic acid during the first year (5mg) is supplied by approximately 900ml human milk or 600ml cows' milk.

(iv) **Vitamin B₆ (pyridoxine)** performs several functions in the metabolism of amino acids. It is concerned with the conversion of tryptophan to nicotinic acid, and is necessary for the formation of the red blood pigment haemoglobin. Vitamin B₆ occurs in a wide variety of foods and thus a deficiency is rare. Very occasionally infants develop convulsions and other disturbances of the

27

nervous system which are cured by doses of vitamin B_6 far in excess of normal intakes. The cause of this apparently increased need for the vitamin is unknown.

Folic acid occurs in many foods, but it is essentially plentiful in liver and green leafy vegetables. The vitamin is easily destroyed by cooking, and significant amounts may be lost in the water used for cooking vegetables.

Folic acid is required for normal blood formation, and a deficiency, which occasionally occurs in pregnant women or after taking certain drugs (anticonvulsants), leads to a characteristic (megaloblastic) form of anaemia.

Vitamin B_{12} is found only in animal products. Liver is the richest source but eggs, cheese, milk, meat and fish have useful amounts. Vitamin B_{12} is required by rapidly dividing cells, such as those in the bone marrow which form blood. A deficiency causes pernicious anaemia and the degeneration of nerve cells. People taking a strictly vegetarian (vegan) diet should take supplementary vitamin $_{12}$.

Biotin is required for the metabolism of fat. It occurs in a wide variety of food – milk, dairy products, cereals, fish, fruit and vegetables. Offal and egg yolk are particularly rich sources. Small amounts are supplied by the bacteria that normally inhabit the large intestine and this source may be sufficient for our needs. A dietary source may therefore not be necessary.

Pantothenic acid plays a central role in fat metabolism. This vitamin is widely distributed in food and a dietary deficiency is unlikely.

Carnitine is a naturally occurring amino acid derivative which plays an important role in the oxidation of fatty acids. Carnitine is not an essential dietary factor for normal adults, but in infants its biosynthesis may be impaired due to the immaturity of certain enzymes.

Breast milk and infant formulas based on cows' milk contain adequate levels of carnitine. However, formulas based on soya or other protein sources contain little or no carnitine. In order to ensure an adequate intake, manufacturers of these non-cows' milk based formulas usually add carnitine to their products to achieve levels similar to those found in breast milk.

It should be borne in mind that cases of gross vitamin deficiencies in the United Kingdom are uncommon. When they do occur, the underlying cause may not be a simple lack of food or the right type of food. The fundamental problem may be a social one, such as an educationally subnormal mother who is unable to appreciate the special dietary needs of a young baby, or the language difficulties experienced by an immigrant mother. These problems require more than giving sound dietary advice, and support from professionals from a variety of disciplines may be needed.

The provision of an adequate intake of nutrients, once solid foods have been introduced at about four months, is ensured by giving the baby a wide range of foods such as meats, dairy produce, fruits, vegetables and cereal products. A diet made up of foods taken from all these groups, without an excessive consumption of foods from any one group, will provide an infant with a satisfactory intake of necessary nutrients.

The daily intakes of nutrients recommended for infants aged 0–2 years are given in Table 3.1.

References

1. Department of Health and Social Security, 1979. Report on Health and Social Subjects No. 15, HMSO, London
2. World Health Organisation, 1985. Technical Report Series 724, Geneva
3. Richie C D and Naismith D J, 1975. A comparison of growth in wholly breast fed infants and in artificially fed infants. Proceedings of the Nutrition Society. Abstracts of Communications 118A
4. Francis D E M, 1986. Nutrition for Children. Blackwell Scientific Publications, Oxford
5. Barltrop D, 1974. Lipid composition and absorption by low birth weight infants. Pediatric Research, 8, 138
6. Jensen C, Buist NRM and Wilson T, 1986. Absorption of individual fatty acids from long chain or medium chain triglycerides in very small infants. American Journal of Clinical Nutrition, 43 745–751
7. Widdowson E M et al, 1975. Body fat of British and Dutch infants. British Medical Journal, 1, 653
8. Department of Health and Social Security, 1980. Artificial feeds for the young infant. HMSO, London
9. Braun O H, 1981. Effect of consumption of human milk and other formulas on intestinal bacterial flora in infants. In: Textbook of Gastroenterology and Nutrition in Infancy, ed Lebenthal E, Raven Press, New York
10. Lee P C, Word K S and Lebenthal E, 1981. Digestibility of starches in infants. In: Textbook of Gastroenterology and Nutrition in Infancy, ed Lebenthal E, Raven Press, New York
11. Heine W, Lenschow U, Drescher U and Wutzke K, 1984. Protein utilisation from baby foods containing starch and dextrin and based on cows' milk. Kinderarztliche Praxis, 9, 428–432
12. Department of Health and Social Security, 1974. Report on Health and Social Subjects No. 9, HMSO, London
13. Wharton B A, 1987. Nutrition and feeding of preterm infants. Report of the Committee on Nutrition of the Preterm Infant (ESPGAN), Blackwell Scientific Publications, Oxford
14. Anon, 1987. Iron deficiency – time for a community campaign? The Lancet, 1, 141–142
15. Addy D P, 1986. Happiness is iron. British Medical Journal, 292, 969–970
16. Aukett M A, Parks Y A, Scott P H and Wharton B A, 1986. Treatment with iron increases weight gain and psychomotor development. Archives of Disease in Childhood, 61, 849–857
17. Carty H, 1988. Brittle or battered. Archives of Disease in Childhood, 63, 350–352
18. Shaw J C L, 1988. Copper deficiency and non-accidental injury. Archives of Disease in Childhood, 63, 448–455
19. Levine R S, 1985. The scientific basis of dental health education. A policy document issued by the Health Education Authority, London
20. Department of Health and Social Security, 1988. Report on Health and Social Subjects No. 32, HMSO, London
21. Taitz L S, 1988. Which children need vitamins? British Medical Journal, 296, 1753–1754
22. Goel K M, Sweet E M, Campbell S et al, 1981. Reduced prevalence of rickets in Asian children in Glasgow. Lancet, ii, 405–407
23. Dunnigan M G, Glekin B M, Henderson J B at al, 1985. Prevention of rickets in Asian children: assessment of the Glasgow campaign. British Medical Journal, 291, 239–242
24. Lammi-Keefe C J and Jensen R G, 1984. Fat soluble vitamins in human milk. Nutrition Reviews, 42, 365–371
25. Aggett P J and Davies N T, 1983. Some nutritional aspects of trace metals. Journal of Inherited Metabolic Disease, 6, Suppl 1, 22–30
26. George D E and Lebenthal E, 1981. Human breast milk in comparison to cows' milk. In: Textbook of Gastroenterology and Nutrition in Infancy, Vol 1, ed Lebenthal E, Raven Press, New York
27. Department of Health and Social Security, 1977. Report on Health and Social Subjects No. 12, HMSO, London
28. Paul A A and Southgate D A T, 1978. McCance and Widdowson's The Composition of Foods, 4th edit., HMSO, London
29. A Report of the Child Health and Nutrition Working Party, 1987. British Dietetic Association.

CHAPTER 4

Breast milk: its composition, advantages and disadvantages

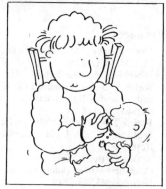

Breast milk has proved its worth over millions of years. Like the milk of every mammal, it is matched to the specific requirements of the growing young, and provides protection against infections.[1]

It is only in the last 100,000 years that man has become a keeper of milk-producing animals, and only in the present century that the use of cows' milk for feeding babies has become widespread, to the extent that in some parts of the world it is considered 'normal'.[2]

Many factors are involved in the mother's decision whether or not to breast feed. Foremost among these are socioeconomic circumstances, age, education and parity. Sadly, it would seem that those who can least afford to buy infant formulas and feeding equipment are those who tend not to breast feed.

Breast development and how milk is made

The mammary glands begin developing in the fetus before the third month of fetal life, originating from the skin.[5] By birth, some primitive duct development has occurred, but it is the rise in ovarian oestrogens during puberty that causes a rapid extension and branching of the duct system, with development of the nipple and areola, and an overall increase in size, mainly due to an increase in fat. Individual breast size does not indicate success or failure to breast feed. Variations in human mammary function are genetic and are related to age. It has been found that there is a steady decline in both milk yield and fat content of milk from older mothers.[5]

During pregnancy, it is likely that the release of human placental lactogen (HPL) stimulates growth of the mammary gland in anticipation of lactation.

Each breast consists of 12 to 20 lobes which are separated by varying amounts of fat. Each lobe is subdivided into lobules which end in milk-secreting glands (alveoli or acini), which receive a rich blood supply.

Secretion of milk is an osmo-regulatory process, and lactose, which is formed in the lumen of the Golgi apparatus of the secretory cell, is the major controlling factor in the production of the aqueous phase of milk and in the determination of milk yield.[6] Lactose is able to set up a potential difference across the cell membrane, and thus keeps the sodium and potassium concentrations lower than they are in blood. Milk is secreted continuously, and is stored in the mammary ducts and alveoli between bouts of suckling.[7]

Differences in composition between preterm and term milk are explained by the probability of an alternative pathway for the secretion of substances from the blood, which involves some leakage of small molecules and ions

30

between milk secreting cells and extracellular fluid (ECF). Thus colostrum and preterm milk are much higher in sodium and chloride, and lower in potassium and lactose, than term milk. During established lactation, the pathway between neighbouring cells is closed.

Milk storage and release

An hour or so after a feed, one-third of the volume of milk for the next feed is already waiting in the distended ducts, and is known as fore milk. The remaining two-thirds is known as the hind milk, and is forced into the milk ducts by contraction of the muscles surrounding each milk gland in response to the 'let-down' reflex. This is a delicately balanced mechanism, and occurs in most women before the tactile stimulus of the baby suckling. Oxytocin is released from the pituitary gland usually three to ten minutes before feeding the baby,[8] and induces contraction of the myofibrils around the alveolar walls, thus squeezing milk into the ducts. A second release of oxytocin also occurs in most women in response to the baby suckling, after which it is released in a pulsatile manner during the feed.[8] Prolactin is also involved, but this is released only in response to direct stimulation of the nipple.

The release of milk in this way can be inhibited by physical and psychological stresses, and women are especially susceptible in the early stages of lactation.

Milk secretion is very much a 'supply and demand' process: more suckling induces more milk via increased prolactin secretion. Induced lactation or adoptive lactation has been well documented[7] and is related to the sucking stimulus of the breast and the release of prolactin.

Colostrum

Colostrum is made by the breasts during late pregnancy. For two to three days its secretion is continued together with milk, which results in a rich yellow mixture.

In composition, it has been thought of as being half-way between the blood which nourished the baby in the uterus and breast milk. It contains much more protein than mature human milk, and this is made up in different proportions. For example, about half of the protein is immunoglobulin (IgA), which forms only about 11 per cent of the total protein in mature milk.[29] Colostrum also contains a large amount of sodium, which is thought to be related to the needs of the baby during a period of very rapid growth. Its pattern of fatty acids is also quite different from that of mature milk.

Due to its high level of protective factors, colostrum is a powerful medicine, able to give the baby some immunity within minutes of his or her entry into the non-uterine, non-sterile world.

Composition of breast milk

Breast milk is a unique food, adapted to nourish the human infant and in particular his brain, which needs derivatives of essential fatty acids (EFA) such as linoleic acid.[14] It also provides antibacterial factors, antibodies and aids to digestion.[1] Table 4.1 shows typical variations in composition.

TABLE 4.1: Composition of mature breast milk:
Range of values to show variations
(Values per 100 ml)

Protein	g	0.95 – 1.20
Fat	g	3.7 – 4.8
Carbohydrate	g	7.1 – 7.8
Energy	kcal	65 – 75
Cholesterol	mg	10 – 23
Vitamin A	μg retinol	40 – 76
Vitamin C	mg	3.1 – 4.5
Thiamin	mg	13 – 21
Riboflavin	mg	31
Nicotinic acid	mg	0.21 – 0.27
Vitamin B_6	μg	5.1 – 7.2
Vitamin B_{12}	μg	0.01
Folic acid	μg	3.1 – 6.2
Biotin	μg	0.13 – 0.72
Pantothenic acid	mg	0.22 – 0.27
Sodium	mg	11 – 20
Potassium	mg	57 – 62
Chloride	mg	35 – 55
Calcium	mg	32 – 36
Magnesium	mg	2.6 – 3.0
Phosphorus	mg	14 – 15
Iron	μg	62 – 93
Copper	μg	37 – 43
Zinc	μg	260 – 330

Breast milk is a living tissue, like blood,[1,6] and indeed contains similar constituents. Its high proportion of lactose (milk sugar) makes it sweet tasting and thus palatable to babies, who show a distinct preference for sweetness[9,10] even when they are born prematurely.[11] In fact taste buds are structurally mature from the 20th week after conception, and saccharin solutions which are injected into amniotic fluid are accepted by the fetus (cited[11]).

About the only thing that is absolutely certain is the variability of the composition of human breast milk from mother to mother, from one stage of lactation to another, and from one feed to another.[3,12,13]

Because of this variability, breast milk may not necessarily be the best sole food for a fast-growing premature infant.

The mother's diet also affects milk composition, especially its content of vitamins, minerals, fatty acids and trace elements. Even so, this is not always significant, except in extreme circumstances. In the same way that mothers in third world countries seem to be resilient to extremely low intakes of vitamins, frank vitamin deficiencies in breast fed babies are surprisingly rare.[13]

Volume of milk produced also varies between mothers, and to some extent is dependent on the frequency of feeds.[3]

Chapter 3, 'An infant's nutritional needs', deals in depth with the fat, protein, carbohydrates, vitamins and minerals which are essential to the infant diet and which are found in breast milk. It is necessary here only to add one or two points.

Fat

Variations in fat content have a profound influence on the energy values of different samples of breast milk. Fat content rises markedly over the first two weeks of lactation and, as it does so, the amounts of phospholipid and cholesterol remain the same or decrease.[18,19]

Within the period of suckling, the fat content changes: at the beginning of a feed it is around 1 to 2 per cent, while towards the end it is around 5 to 7 per cent. Why this should happen is not clear. Visually, there is an obvious change from 'watery' to 'thick' milk. It was formerly believed that a baby initially sucks vigorously in order to satisfy thirst, and then, as the feed becomes more energy dense and the baby becomes satisfied, sucking is less enthusiastic.[20] It was thought that the richer milk was less sweet and therefore less palatable as, with the rise in fat content, the lactose is effectively 'diluted'. However, subsequent studies have shown that babies do not reduce their intake of milk if they are switched from a low fat to a high fat milk,[21,22] and will happily return to the originally suckled breast.[23] Another study showed no indication that a high fat milk acted as a cue to babies to slow or stop feeding.[24]

How babies do control their intake appears to be highly individual. Mothers used to be advised to breast feed for 20 minutes, but in a study from Edinburgh this was found to be inappropriate for the majority of mothers.[25] The majority of babies took most of their feed during the first four minutes on each breast. Nutritive feeding was actually about ten minutes or less, which raises the question of the need for non-nutritive sucking or play at the end of feeding time. It may well be that this is important in establishing a strong mother-infant bond. The lesson to be learned from this study is the highly individual nature of breast feeding: mothers should be encouraged to time their feeds according to their babies' responses.[25] Babies suck in bursts, and it seems that an alert or stimulated baby sucks regardless of whether he is hungry or not.[26]

The pattern of fatty acids also changes as lactation proceeds. Initially, long chain fatty acids predominate: later they decrease, and medium chain fatty acids are more evident.[19,42A] This is also influenced by the mother's weight loss after the birth and by her diet.[27] Mothers in the USA, for example, have more polyunsaturated fatty acids (PUFA) in their milk than UK mothers. The difference reflects the higher PUFA content of the diet of American mothers. This is not necessarily an advantage, as the requirement for vitamin E is increased with increased PUFA.[28] Throughout lactation, the ratio of

PUFA to saturated fatty acids remains constant at about 0.32:1. The cholesterol concentration remains relatively high.

Protein

For many years, the protein content of mature human milk has been assumed to be around 1.2g/100ml.[16] Recent studies, however, have shown that the available protein in breast milk is about half this, i.e. 0.6g/100ml.[19,29]

This discrepancy has arisen partly because of the traditional methods of analysing milk proteins, and partly because it had been assumed that all of them are equally absorbable. It is now thought probable that not all of the whey proteins are nutritionally available.

About 25 per cent of the total nitrogen in breast milk is in the form of amino acids, which can be absorbed immediately. Human milk is unique in this respect.[1]

Taurine and cysteine are present in high concentrations in breast milk, and there is increasing evidence that taurine may be more important than was once thought in the development of the baby.

Carbohydrate

The principal carbohydrate in breast milk is lactose, a disaccharide which, together with other sugars and glycoproteins, comprises about 40 per cent of the energy value. Infants who cannot tolerate it thrive on lactose-free milks. It does, however, seem to play an important role in maintaining the acidity of the gut, and hence the integrity of the gut flora, and in the absorption of calcium.[3,30]

Galactose, one of the monosaccharides making up lactose, appears to be involved in the development of myelin sheaths of the nervous system.[1]

Vitamins

The vitamin content of breast milk from a well nourished mother is usually sufficient to meet the demands of her baby, though there may be exceptions with regard to vitamins D and K.[1,3] The water soluble vitamins in breast milk (B complex and C) reflect levels in the mother's diet and are also related to the time of gestation. Preterm milk, for example, has been shown to be poorer in vitamin B_1 (thiamin), folate and B_6 (pyridoxine).[31]

Megadoses of vitamins are defined as an intake of ten or more times the recommended daily intake (RDA), and are considered unnecessary in an otherwise well-nourished woman.[32] Indeed, with pharmacological doses of some vitamins, there is danger of toxicity.[33,34]

The relatively high concentration of vitamin E in human milk is of interest, and is thought to be associated with its function as a powerful antioxidant for PUFA, especially linoleic acid.[30] Its concentration, however, decreases as lactation progresses.[19]

That wholly breast fed infants rarely develop rickets as a result of vitamin D deficiency has been regarded as proof that breast milk is adequate in this respect.[3] However, vitamin D is normally considered a fat soluble vitamin, and the lipid fraction of breast milk shows a low concentration. It is advisable for breast feeding mothers to ensure that they have a good vitamin D intake, either from the sunshine or from their diet.

In theory, with adequate exposure to sunshine, supplementary vitamin D may not be necessary for breast fed white infants. The question arises because of reports of the appearance of rickets in such babies (cited[35]). A study from the University of Cincinnati Medical Center[35] shows that exposure to sunshine and blood concentrations of 25 hydroxyvitamin D were significantly related in breast fed babies at one, three and six months of age, thus supporting the contention that they may not require vitamin supplements if they have sufficient time in the sunshine. However, great care should be taken to ensure that babies are not over-exposed to the sun, since in adults over-exposure is now believed to play a significant role in skin cancers.

Vitamin D for early post natal life is best obtained from reserves which are laid down during pregnancy, and this lends support to the need for adequacy of maternal vitamin D at this time.

Minerals

The mineral content of breast milk represents about 2g/litre, which is low compared with cows' milk. This is physiologically important, as it results in a lower solute load for the immature kidney[30] – an interesting point in view of the fact that colostrum is very high in sodium. It is thought likely that the infant kidney is more capable of drawing back filtered sodium into the blood than the adult.[17] As the babies mature, sodium balance changes from negative to positive.

The trace elements iron, copper, zinc and manganese, and the minerals calcium and magnesium, are among those which are essential for growth and development. Bioavailability of these is greater from human milk than it is from cows' milk, and it is thought that this is due, at least in part, to the way in which they are bound to membrane proteins in both the lipid and protein fractions.[36]

Breast milk contains the iron-binding protein lactoferrin, which prevents the growth of harmful bacteria. Even so, iron from breast milk is well absorbed[36] as are also zinc and manganese, probably by similar processes involving lactoferrin.[37,38]

Protective factors

Although technology has produced infant formulas which are remarkably near the gross composition of breast milk, one thing which is currently not possible is the addition of the protective factors which are unique to colostrum and to the milks of mammals. A full term human infant is able to suckle within minutes of birth, and thus begins to build up its immunity to disease.

Some of these factors are antibacterial, including **lactoferrin,** which controls the growth of: pathogenic bacteria such as coliforms; yeasts such as *Candida albicans; Streptococcus mutans* which causes dental caries; and other bacteria.[1] The **bifidus factor** encourages the growth of *Lactobacillus bifidus* and an acidic environment, thus further suppressing growth of pathogens.

Lysozyme acts with one of the immunoglobulins (IgA) against *Salmonellae*. **Phagocytic leucocytes** are especially active against *E. coli* and *Candida albicans,* and are especially concentrated in colostrum.

Other antibacterial factors, especially in colostrum, include **lactoperoxidase** and free fatty acids.

Immunoglobulins and **complement proteins** complete the battery of defence mechanisms, the pattern of immunity present in human milk being characteristic of the mother's own immunological experience.

The are several immunoglobulins, of which the predominant one is IgA. It is found in secretions, and is able to form a coating over the mucosa of the baby's alimentary canal and nasal passages. This effectively blocks the passage of large molecules and viruses which would otherwise gain entry.[1] It is also possible that it coats the Eustachian tubes and thus may prevent ear infections. Further, IgA is thought to prevent the development of allergies by blocking sensitising molecules. When IgA is deficient, IgE, which is responsible for immediate hypersensitivity reactions, becomes dominant.

It is thought that breast fed babies may be less likely to develop allergies and infections affecting the gastrointestinal and respiratory tracts (cited[1,15]).

Nutritional status of the mother does not seem to affect these protective factors, though they are affected by duration of gestation, duration of lactation and parity.[39,40,41] Each mother maintains a characteristic level of protective factors. IgA, lactoferrin and lysozyme levels are highest in colostrum and preterm milk.

Human milk would also appear to have antiparasitic activity. *Giardia lamblia* is a common intestinal parasite which can be picked up by people travelling or living in warm climates. It has been observed[42] that breast milk was able to destroy *G. lamblia* by a mechanism which was independent of antibodies, and which involved the production of by-products which were toxic to the parasite, during fat digestion.

All mammalian milk, including breast milk, contains additional hormones, peptides, amino acids and glycoproteins, which may be involved in the development and maturation of the small intestine. In the early postnatal period, the small intestine is immature and relatively susceptible to penetration by harmful agents such as pathogenic bacteria and food antigens. Epidemiological evidence in humans, and laboratory findings in animals, suggest that their milk decreases the incidence of infectious diarrhoea, necrotising enterocolitis, and possibly the development of food allergies. Evidence for the last is suggestive but not conclusive.[42A]

Antibiotic treatment of a breast feeding mother alters the nature of bacterial colonisation within the lactiferous sinuses and nipple.

Growth modulators have only relatively recently been described in breast milk, and may influence nutrient requirements (cited[30]).

Effect of extended lactation on composition

When lactation proceeds for more than six months, the composition of breast milk undergoes some considerable changes in vitamin and mineral content.[43] This is related to the onset of weaning and the decrease in frequency of breast feeding. Zinc and calcium content show decreases which are related to the frequency of feeding, and magnesium concentration also decreases but very much more slowly.

During weaning, the mammary glands undergo considerable changes in their secretory function, due to depletion of fat and an increase in connective tissue. The decrease in mineral concentration could reflect a gradual involution of the mammary gland as a result of reducing the frequency of breast feeding. Vitamins B_6 and C concentrations also decrease, but folate remains unchanged. If breast feeding is terminated abruptly, there appears to be an increase in fat, protein, sodium and chloride, which is probably due to increasing transport by the paracellular pathway.[2]

When lactation continues for a year or more, the fat content decreases to a constant level.[44]

Lactation and the mother's diet

It is still not clear how lactation in humans is controlled and regulated. For example, is milk production governed by the mother's diet, by the demands of her breast fed infant, or by both?

In theory it should be easy to answer this, by giving supplements to breast feeding women to see if milk output increases, and then reducing energy intake in well nourished mothers to see if milk output is compromised. In practice, however, it does not work out as one might expect.

The volume of milk produced by nutritionally depleted mothers may be reduced to a limited extent, but the gross composition remains remarkably constant.[45]

Studies which have examined the dietary intakes of exclusively breast feeding mothers suggest that there are enormous individual variations not only in food intakes, but also in the metabolic adaptations which take place during lactation in order to provide sufficient milk, and hence in the mothers' ability to breast feed adequately for varying lengths of time, say from 2½ months to 15 months.[46,47,48,49] A voluntary and severe 'reducing' diet, however, could have an adverse though delayed effect, and is not recommended.[47]

Studies such as these shed doubt on the old idea that breast feeding mothers need to 'eat for two'. It may be that current RDA's are too high in energy intake (calories), and do not take into account the adaptations which the body makes in order to 'save' calories for milk production.[46,50] Such changes are stimulated by suckling, and the mother who has difficulty in feeding is encouraged to feed more frequently.[46] The mother's appetite is probably the best guide, and she should be advised how to choose a well balanced diet.

Fluid requirements during lactation

Fluid intake during lactation is very variable between mothers, so that there are no hard and fast rules about drinking more. Prolactin itself appears to have an antidiuretic, water-sparing effect, in order to retain sodium and water.[7]

37

In practice, some women find that they get thirsty while breast feeding, and this is their best guide to fluid requirements. It is also thought that a drink just before or during a feed is relaxing. Neither quantity nor quality of milk is improved by forcing a mother to drink more than she wants to.

Adequacy of lactation

Most full term infants obtain enough nutrients in the right proportions from their mothers' milk, so that they are able to grow at the rate determined by their genetic potential.[15] But babies vary enormously in their intakes of milk. At two months of age, the intakes of breast fed infants have been seen to range from 445 to 1235ml daily (cited[15]), and these differences could not be accounted for in terms of the babies' body weights.

Most estimates of breast milk requirements have been based on the volumes necessary to satisfy energy needs, but it is now thought that these may be too generous.[13,15] Such values are only commensurate with above-average lactational capacities.[13]

At present it is thought that the baby is the best judge of what he needs, and that mothers should be encouraged to follow their own instincts, provided that the baby is growing well and developing normally.[13]

Babies who are not being adequately breast fed appear to be of two types. One type is fretful and has short, frequent feeds, which are often associated with colic and vomiting. The other type appears to be 'contented', is sleepy, and has long intervals between feeds.[51]

Hypernatraemia is not something which one would immediately consider as a possible reason for failing to thrive at the breast, but some samples of breast milk have been shown to have abnormally high levels of sodium, resulting in dehydration and an ill baby.[52,80,81]

The nutritional quality of breast milk also needs to be considered in relation to the health and customs of the mother. Beriberi has been reported in the baby of a thiamin deficient mother; vitamin B_{12} deficiency in a baby whose mother was a strict vegan; and mineral and vitamin deficiencies in premature babies.[53] Breast milk is not suitable for babies who are born with galactosaemia or lactose intolerance.

Good body growth is important not only for its own sake in producing a healthy child, but also for brain growth. The brain growth spurt begins in mid-pregnancy and continues well into the second year of life.[54] Undernutrition at this time may be expected to affect brain growth, and the capacity for subsequent recovery is not known. It is certainly true that most previously undernourished children are poor achievers in later life, and Prof John Dobbing warns about being overcautious in the avoidance of overfeeding a child.[54]

The nutritional and protective benefits of breast milk are well recognised. But enthusiasm for its promotion should not obscure the fact that not all breast fed babies receive an adequate supply.[52] In addition, one has to be realistic in recognising occasions when breast milk is not the perfect food.[53] Dogmatic statements about the length of time to breast feed, and the introduction of mixed feeding, should therefore be avoided.

Drugs in breast milk

Almost any drug which a breast feeding mother may take, be it for medical, social or other reasons, is excreted via her milk, though the extent of this is dependent on the drug itself, the rate at which it is metabolised, and the composition of the milk.[53,55] Ideally, nursing mothers should take no drugs while breast feeding, but in some instances drugs cannot be avoided. There may be some concern for the baby if drugs are used for a long time, except for drugs which are not systemically active by mouth in the infant, e.g. insulin excreted by diabetic mothers.

It has been long known that nicotine is excreted in the breast milk of mothers who smoke.[56] What is not clear is whether the baby receives most nicotine from the milk, or by inhaling it from the atmosphere. Mothers who smoke tend not to breast feed their babies, but those who breast feed may find that smoking affects their success in maintaining lactation.[57]

Alcohol is excreted in breast milk, but moderate maternal alcohol consumption has not been known to affect the baby adversely.[30]

Of more recent concern has been the finding that some environmental pollutants become concentrated in the food chain, are stored in adipose tissue, and then excreted in breast milk. To date, however, there have been no reports of illness in breast fed babies due to these residues.[53]

Although more mothers may be willing to breast feed now, some 20 to 40 per cent may be disappointed by not producing sufficient milk. A study from Finland tested a drug, sulpiride, which stimulates the production of prolactin, and which resulted in higher milk yields from most of the women taking part.[58]

Why breast feed?

Probably the best answer to the question 'Why breast feed?' is 'because Nature intended it'. Indeed, in the present climate of 'no artificial additives', 'pure and natural', 'home grown' and 'organic', that answer may be readily acceptable.[59] Other claims that have been made over the years in favour of breast feeding, however, have not all survived scientific scrutiny.

A mother who does not breast feed is just as capable of being a good and loving mother as one who does. It is not the business of professional advisers to approve or disapprove of a woman's decision, but rather to make her aware of the facts, and give her the support she needs in whatever choice she makes.

The ability of a woman to breast feed successfully, according to some authorities, is determined during pregnancy, and is related to her weight before pregnancy and her weight gain during it. One study concluded that the only difference between 'successful' and 'unsuccessful' breast feeders was the amount of weight gained during pregnancy. If this was 5kg or less, the mothers experienced difficulties.[60]

Coronary heart disease. It has been claimed that the high cholesterol content of breast milk somehow initiates a metabolic pathway for cholesterol, which prevents its accumulation and association with arterial disease later on.[61] However, further studies give no support to this.[62]

Intelligence. It has been suggested that breast feeding and early skin-to-skin contact is associated with a higher level of intelligence, especially in boys (cited[1]). A further study, which followed breast fed children up to the age of five, found that if there were any associations of this kind, they were very small.[63] Other factors were more important, such as socioeconomic status, maternal age and education.

Avoiding obesity. Certainly there is no risk of over-concentrated feeds with breast feeding, but now that highly modified, low solute infant formulas are widely available, there is no reason to believe that bottle fed babies will be fatter than breast fed babies.[59] It is no longer believed that early feeding practices determine body weight at six weeks or six months. More important is birth weight and feeding style. A study from the USA noticed that heavier infants suck more vigorously, and take in more calories from each feed, than do lighter infants.[64] It is certainly easier to obtain milk from a bottle than from the breast.

Allergies. Because of the effectiveness of IgA, especially in colostrum, it is often said that even if a mother can breast feed for a minimum of two weeks, she will confer at least some protection on her baby. For the infant who is likely to be atopic, continuation of breast feeding is probably sensible, as the development of typical atopic features such as rhinitis, bronchitis, gastrointestinal and respiratory upsets, asthma, otitis media and eczema, tend to be reduced with breast feeding (cited[15]). However, a study of over 13,000 children showed no effect of breast feeding on the incidence of bronchitis or lower respiratory disease. It did have a marginal effect on reducing the incidence of gastrointestinal disease.[65]

The risk of developing allergy to milk proteins is greatest in infancy, and most infants develop antibodies to beta lactoglobulin (cited[15]). In some instances, breast fed babies may be sensitised to cows' milk protein via their mothers' milk, and symptoms like colic may develop. Avoidance of cows' milk products by the mother for the period of breast feeding may help to alleviate symptoms in the baby, but this is not always a certain cure.[66]

It is also possible that breast milk contains protective features for the breast itself. Prof Dobbing asks whether breast abscess might be even more common without the immunity-conferring properties of milk.[59]

Dental caries. It is sometimes said that breast fed babies are less susceptible to dental caries than bottle fed babies, but evidence one way or the other is not satisfactory.

If a baby is allowed to fall asleep at his mother's breast, e.g. during night time feeding, acid fermentation of sugars can begin, because milk is not being cleared quickly from the mouth, as in normal feeding.[68] Obviously not all babies who feed at night will develop dental caries, but there is no way of finding out which are more at risk than others.

Emotional aspects. There is more to breast feeding, say the enthusiasts, than the provision of nutrients, bacterial flora, and antiinfective and antiallergic factors.[15]

Breast feeding is thought to promote bonding between mother and child, especially if contact between them is almost immediate after the birth. The relationship between a mother and her breast fed child is thought to be so different from that between a mother and her bottle fed child, that subsequent feeding patterns and behaviour might be affected (cited[15]).

There is no real evidence for this, one way or the other.[59] For some mothers, breast feeding may even have an adverse effect on the relationship with the baby. What is important is the method of feeding with which the mother feels most comfortable. Experience suggests, however, that breast feeding can be rewarding and satisfying for most mothers.

Sudden infant death

Many hypotheses have been put forward as to the cause of sudden death in babies, some of which are nutritional in origin. It was suggested at one time, for example, that cot deaths are more common in bottle fed babies, possibly due to the accidental inhalation of cows' milk protein,[69] but this is not now thought to be the case. Some breast fed babies do die suddenly and unexpectedly, and no clear pattern seems to have emerged which relates this tragic occurrence with the method of feeding.

Low birth weight, prematurity, diarrhoea and feeding difficulties are known risk factors.[71] Many babies who suffer cot death are not entirely symptom free. Perhaps some deaths could be prevented by improved parental awareness of symptoms such as overheating, abnormal crying, irritability, sleepiness, snuffles, cough, diarrhoea and vomiting, and also by better medical care. It is difficult for parents to know when such apparently minor symptoms are important, but it would seem that a combination of these together with an over-warm, oppressive atmosphere could turn into potential danger.[70]

It remains a mystery whether there is an underlying condition which acts as a trigger or is the actual cause of death, or whether genetic elements are involved.[72] What is felt to be important is that the mother should not be saddled with a feeling of guilt that she has not fed her baby correctly, and that this was the cause of her loss.[59]

The question of breast cancer

In the past, women have been told that breast feeding may protect them from developing breast cancer, but despite extensive studies there appears to be no clear-cut relationship. A large study from Norway gave the overall impression that breast feeding is not associated with a risk of cancer of the breast or of any other common kind of cancer.[73]

What does seem to matter is the age at which a woman has her first child. The older the mother, the greater the risk.[74] Other factors which seem to be involved are obesity, lack of exercise, and dietary fat (cited[75]).

Breast feeding as a natural contraceptive

Breast feeding has long been known to inhibit ovulation by maintaining high prolactin levels, and so to reduce the likelihood of conception. However, because women vary so much, it is not a completely reliable method of contraception for an individual, particularly a well nourished one. Frequency of suckling, time between feeds, and the total duration of suckling are all important factors in maintaining infertility.[76] Return of ovulation, and hence the risk of pregnancy, is much higher when breast feeding is reduced to 60 minutes a day, i.e. when other feeds are being given to the baby.[77]

Weight loss after birth

It is often said that breast feeding results in the mother's quickly returning to her 'normal' pre-pregnancy weight, but this is hard to substantiate.

Naismith found that women who gained the most weight during pregnancy tended to *lose* the most weight, and to eat less, during lactation. Those who gained less during pregnancy ate more, and lost less weight, during lactation.[78]

Postnatal weight loss seems to vary from woman to woman. Some seem able to conserve their own energy, and to use it to subsidise milk production.[47] This efficient use of energy, which could be due to inhibition of brown fat activity and of non-shivering thermogenesis, may explain why some breast feeding women simply cannot lose weight. Although they may complain of being hungry, they may still eat too much to burn up. Those who breast feed and 'eat for two' may find it hard to lose weight.[47]

A study from Aberdeen concluded that weight loss, and the characteristics of body fat, are similar in lactating and non-lactating women during the first five to six weeks postnatally.[79]

Summary

Most health professionals are agreed that breast feeding should be promoted, since it is a natural continuation of pregnancy and delivery, and is certainly the least expensive option. However, not all the arguments that have been put forward in the past for its promotion stand up to more recent scientific scrutiny, and in-depth investigations have destroyed some of the myths and mystery surrounding breast feeding.

In balance, experience would suggest that breast feeding is satisfying and rewarding for most mothers, and perhaps for this reason alone they deserve every encouragement and support.

References

1. Whittlestone W G, 1983. A Foundation of Preventive Medicine. Nutrition and Health, **1**, (3/4) 133–141
2. Jelliffe E F P, 1976. Maternal Nutrition and Lactation. In: Breast Feeding and the Mother, Ciba Foundation Symposium 45, 119–143
3. DHSS, 1988. Present Day Practice in Infant Feeding. Third Report. Report on Health and Social Subjects No. 32, HMSO
5. Hytten F E, 1976. The Physiology of Lactation. In: Symposium Issue on Breast Feeding. Journal of Human Nutrition, **30**, (4), 225–232
6. Bisbee, C A, 1981. Prolactin Effects on Ion Transport across Cultured Mouse Mammary Epithelium. American Journal of Physiology, **240**, C110–C115
7. Peaker M, 1976. Physiology of Lactation. In: Breast Feeding and the Mother. Ciba Foundation Symposium 45, 87–101
8. McNeilly S A, Robinson I C A, Houston M J and Howie P, 1983. Release of Oxytocin and Prolactin in Response to Suckling. British Medical Journal, **286**, (Jan 22nd), 257–259

9. Editorial, 1969. Infants' Sweet Tooth. Journal of the American Medical Association, **55**, 458

10. Desor J A, 1973. Taste and Acceptance of Sugars by Human Infants. Journal of Comparative Physiology and Psychology, **84**, (3), 496–501

11. Tatzer E, Schubert M T, Timischl W and Simbruner G, 1985. Discrimination of Taste and Preference for Sweet in Premature Babies. Early Human Development, **12**, 23–30

12. Hibberd C M, Brooke O G, Carter N D et al, 1982. Variation in the Composition of Breast Milk during the First Five Weeks of Lactation: Implications for the Feeding of Preterm Infants. Archives of Disease in Childhood, **57**, 658–662

13. Whitehead R G, 1983. Nutritional Aspects of Human Lactation. Lancet, **i**, 167–169

14. Crawford M, 1983. The Role of Lipids in Early Development, Pregnancy, Oral Contraception and Lactation. Journal of Obstetrics and Gynaecology, **3**, (Supp. 2), S47

15. Cockburn F, 1983. Milk Composition – the Infant Human Diet. In: Symposium on Milk Composition and its Manipulation. Proceedings of the Nutrition Society, **42**, (3), 361–373

16. DHSS, 1977. The Composition of Mature Human Milk. Report on Health and Social Subjects No. 12. HMSO

17. DHSS, 1980. Artificial Feeds for the Young Infant. Report on Health and Social Subjects No. 18. HMSO

18. Changes with Time and the Lipids of Human Milk, 1984. Nutrition Reviews, **42**, (1), 12–13

19. Harzer G, Hang M and Bindels J G, 1986. Biochemistry of Maternal Milk in Early Lactation. Symposium on Fundamental Considerations in Infant Feeding. Human Nutrition: Applied Nutrition Supp, **40A**, 11–18

20. Hall B, 1975. Changing Composition of Human Milk and Early Development of Appetite Control. Lancet, **i**, 779-781

21. Woolridge M W at al, 1980. Does a Change in the Composition of Human Milk Affect Sucking Patterns and Milk Intake? Lancet, **ii**, (8207), 1292–4

22. Bezerra V L, 1982. Correlation between Changeable Human Milk Constituents and Milk Intake in Breast Fed Infants. Journal of Pediatrics, **101**, (1), 80–83

23. Drewett R, 1982. Returning to the Suckled Breast: a Further Test of Hall's Hypothesis. Early Human Development, **7**, 161–163

24. Nysenbaum A N and Smart J L, 1982. Sucking Behaviour and Milk Intake of Neonates in Relation to Milk Fat Content. Early Human Development, **6**, 205–213

25. Howie P W, Houston M J, Cook A et al, 1981. How Long should a Breast Feed Last? Early Human Development, **5**, 71–77

26. Kaye H, 1967. Infant Sucking Behaviour and its Modifications. Advances in Child Development and Behaviour, **3**, 1–52

27. Chappell J E, Claudinin M T and Kearney-Volpe C, 1985. Trans Fatty Acids in Human Milk Lipids: Influence of Maternal Diet and Weight Loss. American Journal of Clinical Nutrition, **42**, 49–56

28. Jansson L, Akesson B and Holmberg L, 1981. Vitamin E and Fatty Acid Composition of Human Milk. American Journal of Clinical Nutrition, **34**, 8–13

29. val Woelderen B F, 1987. Changing Insight into Human Milk Proteins: Some Implications. Nutrition Abstracts and Reviews, **57**, (3), 129–134

30. Hambraeus L, 1984. Human Milk Composition. Nutrition Abstracts and Reviews, **54**, (4), 219–236

31. Ford J E, Zechalko A, Murphy J and Brooke O G, 1983. Comparison of the B Vitamin Composition of Milk from Mothers of Pre-Term and Term Babies. Archives of Disease in Childhood, **58**, 367–372

32. Anderson D M and Pitard W B, 1985. Vitamin E and C Concentrations in Human Milk with Maternal Megadosing: a Case Report. Journal of the American Dietetic Association, **85**, (6), 715–717

33. Vitamin B$_6$ Toxicity: a New Megavitamin Syndrome, 1984. Nutrition Reviews, **42**, (2), 44–46

34. Sensory Neuropathy from Megadoses of Pyridoxine, 1984. Nutrition Reviews, **42**, (2), 49–51

35. Specker B and Tsang R C, 1987. Cyclical Serum 25 Hydroxyvitamin D Concentrations Paralleling Sunshine Exposure in Exclusively Breast Fed Infants. Journal of Pediatrics, **110**, (5), 744–747

36. Fransson G B and Lonnerdal B, 1984. Iron, Copper, Zinc, Calcium and Magnesium in Human Milk Fat. American Journal of Clinical Nutrition, **39**, 185–189
37. Personal Communication
38. Bioavailability of Milk Zinc in Infants, 1984. Nutrition Reviews, **42**, 220–222
39. Banked Milk is Low in Immunologically Protective Proteins, 1987. Nutrition Reviews, **45**, (2), 44–46
40. Prentice A, Prentice A M, Cole T J and Whitehead R G, 1983. Determinants of Variations in Breast Milk Protective Factor Concentrations of Rural Gambian Mothers. Archives of Disease in Childhood, **58**, 518–522
41. Differences Between the Immunology of Term and Preterm Milk, 1984. Nutrition Reviews, **41**, (8), 237–238
42. Products of Lipolysis in Human Milk Destroy Parasites, 1987. Nutrition Reviews, **45**, (8), 236–238
42A. Sheard N F, 1988. The Role of Breast Milk in the Development of the Gastrointestinal Tract. Nutrition Reviews, **46**, (1), 1–8
43. Karra M V, Udipi S A, Kirksey A and Roepke J, 1986. Changes in Specific Nutrients in Breast Milk during Extended Lactation. American Journal of Clinical Nutrition, **43**, (April), 495–503
44. Kon S K and Mawson E H, 1950. Human Milk. Special Report Series of the Medical Research Council, No. 269. HMSO
45. Jelliffe D B and Jelliffe E F P, 1978. The Volume and Composition of Human Milk in Poorly Nourished Communities: a Review. American Journal of Clinical Nutrition, **31**, 492–515
46. Illingworth P, 1985. Feeding Children. Symposium by the McCarrison Society, Scottish Group, October 5th
47. Energy Intake and Lactational Performance in Women, 1987. Nutrition Reviews, **45**, (1), 12–14
48. Butte N F, 1984. Effect of Maternal Diet and Body Composition on Lactational Performance. American Journal of Clinical Nutrition, **39**, 296–306
49. Adequacy of Lactation in Well Nourished Mothers, 1984. Nutrition Reviews, **42**, (1), 8–9
50. Stuff J, Garza C, Boutte C et al, 1986. Sources of Variance in Milk and Caloric Intakes in Breast Fed Infants: Implications for Lactation Study Design and Interpretation. American Journal of Clinical Nutrition, **43**, (March), 361–366
51. Davies D P, 1979. Is Inadequate Breast Feeding an Important Cause of Failure to Thrive? Lancet, **ii**, 238
52. Rowland T W, Zori R T, Lafleur W A and Reiter E O, 1982. Malnutrition and Hypernatraemic Dehydration in Breast Fed Infants. Journal of the American Medical Association, **247**, (7), 1016–1017
53. Coveney J, 1985. Is Breast Milk the Best Food for All Infants? Human Nutrition: Applied Nutrition, **39A**, (3), 179–188
54. Dobbing J, 1984. Infant Nutrition and Late Achievement. Nutrition Reviews, **42**, (1), 1–7
55. Wilson J T, 1983. Contamination of Human Milk by Drugs and Chemicals. Nutrition and Health, **2**, (3/4), 191–201
56. Woodward A, Grgurinovich N and Ryan P, 1986. Breast Feeding and Smoking Hygiene. Journal of Epidemiological and Community Health, **40**, 309–315
57. Lyon A J, 1983. Effects of Smoking on Breast Feeding. Archives of Disease in Childhood, **58**, 378–380
58. Ylikorkala O et al, 1982. Sulpiride Improves Inadequate Lactation. British Medical Journal, **285**, (6337), 249–251
59. Dobbing J, 1984. Breast is Best – Isn't It? In: Health Hazards of Milk. Ed. Freed D L J, Publ. Bailliere Tindall
60. Naismith D J and Ritchie C D, 1975. The Effect of Breast Feeding and Artificial Feeding on Body Weights, Skinfold Measurements and Food Intakes of 42 Primiparous Women. Proceedings of the Nutrition Society, **34**, (3), 116A
61. Marmot M G, Page C M, Atkins E and Douglas J W B, 1980. Effects of Breast Feeding on Plasma Cholesterol and Weight in Young Adults. Journal of Epidemiological and Community Health, **34**, 164–167

62. Burr M L, Beasley W H and Fisher C B, 1984. Breast Feeding, Maternal Smoking and Early Atheroma. European Heart Journal, 5, 588–591
63. Taylor B and Wadsworth J, 1984. Breast Feeding and Child Development at Five Years. Developmental Medicine and Child Neurology, 26, 73–80
64. Agras W S, Karaemer H C, Berkowitz R I et al, 1987. Does a Vigorous Feeding Style Influence Early Development of Obesity? Journal of Pediatrics, 110, (5), 799–804
65. Taylor B, Wadsworth J, Golding J and Butte N, 1982. Breast Feeding, Bronchitis and Admissions for Lower Respiratory Illness and Gastro-Enteritis during the First Five Years. Lancet, i, (8283), 1227–1229
66. Lake A M, Whitington P F and Hamilton S R, 1982. Dietary Protein Induced Colitis in Breast Fed Infants. Journal of Pediatrics, 101, (6), 906–910
68. Farne M P, 1984. Nursing Caries. Journal of Nutrition Education, 16, (4), 158
69. Emery J L, 1984. Sudden Infant Deaths: Are We Asking the Right Questions? Modern Medicine, 29, (10), 9–10
70. Barrie H, 1983. What You Should Know about SIDS. World Medicine, 18, (19), 38–40
71. Simpson H, 1983. Sudden Infant Death. Update, 26, (11), 1951–1959
72. Bain A D, 1981. Sudden Infant Death Syndrome. The Practitioner, 225, 319–325
73. Kvale G and Hench I, 1987. Lactation and Cancer Risk: Is there a Relation Specific to Breast Cancer? Journal of Epidemiology and Community Health, 42, 30–37
74. Short R V, 1976. Discussion on Lactation Infertility. In: Breast Feeding and the Mother, Ciba Foundation Symposium 45, 73–86
75. Pariza M W, 1987. Dietary Fat, Calorie Restriction, Ad Libitum Feeding and Cancer Risk. Nutrition Reviews, 45, (1), 1–7
76. Gross B A and Eastman C J, 1983. Effect of Breast Feeding Status on Prolactin Secretion and Resumption of Menstruation. The Medical Journal of Australia, 1, 313–317
77. Dewart P J and Loudon N B, 1987. Contraception and Lactation. Midwife, Health Visitor and Community Nurse, 23, (8), 333–337
78. Naismith D J, 1980. Maternal Nutrition and the Outcome of Pregnancy – a Critical Appraisal. From: Symposium on Nutrition of the Mother and Child. Proceedings of the Nutrition Society, 39, (1), 1–11
79. Personal Communication
80. Clarke T et al, 1979. Hypernatraemic Dehydration resulting from Inadequate Breast Feeding. Pediatrics, 63, 931-932
81. Ernst J A, Wynn R J and Schreiner R L, 1981. Starvation with Hypernatraemic Dehydration in Two Breast Fed Infants. Journal of the American Dietetic Association, 1981, 79, 126–130

CHAPTER 5

Why women choose not to breast feed

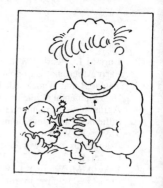

Many health professionals are disappointed that the surge in popularity of breast feeding in Britain in the latter half of the 1970's, has not continued into the 1980's. In fact, two reports from the Office of Population Censuses & Surveys show a slight fall between 1980 and 1985, a tendency which is rather surprising. There are other signs, too, that there will be a decline in coming years.[1] (Fig 5.1)

In spite of research results continually confirming the tangible benefits of breast feeding, and decades of official and professional endorsement of it,[2,3,4,5] it would appear that Britain is predominantly a bottle feeding nation. Only 64 per cent of our babies are ever put to the breast, and this figure rapidly declines as the baby gets older.

At four weeks the majority are at best only partly breast fed; by six weeks the position at birth has practically reversed, with 61 per cent exclusively bottle fed; and by four months, this figure has risen to 74 per cent. At nine months, only 12 per cent of mothers continue to breast feed.[1] (Fig 5.1)

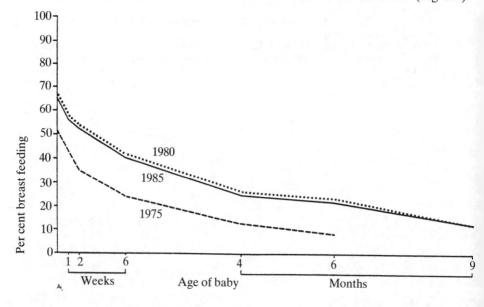

Fig 5.1: Proportions of infants being breast fed in the first 9 months: England and Wales

Mothers breast feeding for less than six weeks have been defined for research purposes as failed breast feeders,[6] and this would apply to about 40 per cent of mothers who now start breast feeding.

So what is going wrong? Why does one mother in three not attempt to breast feed, and why do the others give up so quickly?

One factor is the social expectations of breast feeding and its duration. Bottle feeding is often seen as the norm, and breast feeding as something which only certain people can do, and which in any case will last only for a few weeks. The launch of the 1988 DHSS report on infant feeding was heralded by a headline in *The Times*: 'Report encourages women to breast feed for one year.' This seemed shocking to some and normal to others, although it is in fact a misleading quotation of the Department of Health's Recommendation 14 on weaning.[7] In other countries where there is no alternative to breast feeding, it is normal to breast feed for two years or more, and this can be justified on biological and nutritional grounds.

In the UK, the mother who is most likely to breast feed her first baby, and to continue for the longest period of time, is over 25 years of age, has been educated past the age of 18, comes from a high social class, and lives in the South-East of England.[1] Yet this does not explain why she is likely to choose breast feeding, nor why the very young Scottish mother, with no husband and little education, is likely to opt for bottle feeding.

Clear as these socio-economic indicators are, one must conclude that rather than having a direct effect, they simply reflect the complex factors in a mother's background and environment, such as her attitudes, beliefs and experience, and those of her partner, mother and friends.[8]

Nearly one third of first-time mothers have already decided on their feeding method before becoming pregnant, and most of the remainder decide early on in pregnancy. The experience of feeding the first baby has a major influence on how the next baby is fed. Since so many mothers give up early with their first child,[1] breast feeding becomes somewhat less likely with each subsequent child.

It seems obvious that while established breast feeding can be said to be easy and convenient for the mother, many women who want to establish it find it difficult, frustrating and sometimes even painful. There are several recurrent reasons given by women who cease to breast feed after an initial attempt.[9,10]

Insufficient milk is the most common reason given for stopping during the first four months, and in many ways it is the most tragic. It can be caused by mothers taking inadequate food (Calories) or dieting. A hungry baby should be given more frequent feeds from the breast to increase the milk supply, since a positive feedback mechanism works to achieve this. While it may seem more logical to offer top-up feeds, or to breast feed less frequently, this can only lead to a drop in milk production.

In Western countries, mothers often lack confidence in their ability to sustain their babies totally in the first months. There are no dials on their bras saying 'empty', 'full', or 'baby has taken four ounces'. They may therefore find it hard to believe that this apparently haphazard and relatively invisible process can possibly work. Anxiety, and lack of satisfaction and confidence in the whole process, may interfere with let-down and milk production. This could lead indirectly to insufficient milk. Encouragement and really positive support are needed to prevent this.

Thin milk may also be given as a reason for giving up. Most people know very little about milk. They have probably never considered that each species produces its own type of milk, varying greatly in thickness and colour because of its individual composition, which in turn is governed by the needs of the infant. Although we all know what cows' milk looks like, few people have seen human milk in any quantity. It does look thinner, it is a bluish white, and unlike cows' milk it does not adhere to the sides of glass containers.

Sore nipples can be extremely painful and distressing. This condition may be caused by poor attachment to the breast, a problem which may arise because the baby has become used to a bottle teat. Some babies are simply over-enthusiastic suckers.

Poor sucking is another reason often given for abandoning breast feeding. Support, combined with well informed and sympathetic guidance, is needed to overcome these problems, since the easy option of formula milk will offer rapid relief. A woman with one or two inverted nipples could lose confidence if a fuss is made during pregnancy. However, there is not normally a problem once feeding begins, although this too has been given as a reason for stopping.[10]

Return to work. Although this is a reason often given for ceasing to breast feed, it would seem to be more an excuse than a reality. The 1988 DHSS report *Present Day Practice in Infant Feeding* states (3.12.1): 'A woman's intention to return to paid work soon after having a baby does not seem to be a major influence on her choice of method of feeding.'

The 1985 OPCS survey showed that a minority (11 per cent) of women returned to work within five months of having a baby, and 21 per cent had returned within nine months, most to part-time work. Many mothers breast fed until they returned to work; also, mothers who returned to work early were just as likely to have breast fed before they started work as mothers who did not do paid work when their babies were very young.

A study in the United States showed that good nursery facilities hastened the return to work by hospital staff after maternity leave, and produced a longer duration of breast feeding. On the maternity ward, a much more effective and influential impression of breast feeding was given to the mothers.[11]

Inconsistent advice on feeding methods in general, from health professionals, family, friends, advertising and the media, can confuse mothers. Emphasising too strongly the benefits of breast feeding can offend mothers who have decided to bottle feed, or who have failed to breast feed. Many health professionals are very sensitive to this, and play down the differences between different methods. By the time the relevant ante-natal classes are held, most parents have already decided on their choice of feeding method, and it is too late to influence their decision. It is therefore essential that bottle feeding procedures are discussed.

In a study in Birmingham, 30 per cent of mothers were failed breast feeders, and many of them felt angry and frustrated that they had been unsuccessful. They felt they had been given too much conflicting advice, and asked for clear, simple guidance in the early days, for more in-depth explanation of the physiology of breast feeding, and for a demonstration of breast feeding in the ante-natal stage.[6]

It seems that although mothers and fathers may feel relatively well prepared for the dramatic events of labour, we have neglected to prepare them for the less dramatic, but none the less skilful art of breast feeding. Having a clear policy on breast feeding, so that health professionals are consistent in their advice, has improved breast feeding rates in certain areas.[12] This is particularly important since inconsistent advice on specific feeding problems on the ward may be further confused by the large number of staff employed.

Ideally, perhaps there should be lactation sisters or infant feeding advisers for every ward, or at least for every hospital. Greater continuity of care between health professionals concerned with mother and baby was recommended by COMA, and is one of the ways in which the importance of the role of the professionals is endorsed in its report.[1] UNICEF and WHO have issued a statement that:

'Every family has a right to know that the best protection against both infection and incorrect nutrition is breast feeding for the first four to six months. Other foods should then be added, but breast milk is the best food a child will ever have, and breast feeding should continue well into the second year of life.'[13]

The time taken to breast feed is a major reason for stopping between the first week and the fourth month.[10] Babies need to suck for comfort as well as nutrition, and breast feeding takes longer because the milk flow is low at the end of a feed. On the other hand, a teat with larger holes can be fitted to a bottle of formula milk to speed up the whole process.

Inconvenience is another reason for abandoning breast feeding, and some mothers feel that the bottle seems easier. In many ways this could well be true, even in hospital. In some maternity wards, ready-prepared bottles are available free, and the temptation to have a good night's sleep after a tiring labour, painful stitches, Caesarian section or general exhaustion, is easy to imagine. Rooming-in of babies makes demand feeding easier, leading to successful lactation, and flexibility is desirable in the running of wards.

Yet inconvenience can work both ways. Once the free ready-to-feed formula is no longer around, preparing the feeds can become a chore. A first-time mother will not necessarily know how many bottles to make up in advance, or indeed if it is acceptable to do this. What happens to the inexperienced or immature mother if she runs out of formula milk or cash with which to buy it?

Bottle feeding incurs a cost while breast milk is free, yet poorer mothers still tend to choose bottle feeding. Long journeys on public transport, shopping trips and days out are all factors which affect the decision whether to breast or bottle feed. A mother's personal feelings, and the attitudes of the general public, also play an influential role in the issue of breast feeding in public places.

Many mothers and potential mothers view the idea of breast feeding with distaste. It is a very personal and physical act, and breast feeding women may be surprised at the parasexual feelings that suckling may arouse in them – feelings which are rarely discussed, and which they may not be able to accept.[8] Social class differences in attitudes to sex, personal modesty and so on, are well established, and these may account for much of the social class variation in feeding choice. Fathers may feel that they have been displaced, and be unwilling to 'share' the mother now that her pregnancy is over.

Breast feeding has failed to gain complete social acceptance as the 'normal' way of feeding babies, and the DHSS report urges that mothers should feel free to feed their babies wherever the need arises. It is difficult, however, to envisage this 'ideal' state of affairs until the general public has been re-educated in its attitudes. One in three mothers has experienced problems in finding places to feed her baby in public.[1] Mothers are still asked to leave shops, restaurants and libraries while in the middle of breast feeding, and they are embarrassed and humiliated by the experience. Alternatively they may be asked to go and sit in the lavatory. Baby care facilities which are separate from adult lavatories are now regarded as necessary. The international airport sign for these facilities is a baby's bottle, but the new National Baby Care symbol is more encouraging to breast feeders while still being appropriate to bottle feeders (Fig 5.2)

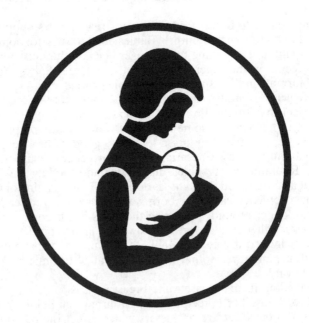

Fig 5.2: The National Baby Care symbol denotes facilities for baby feeding and changing

Illness of the mother is quoted by eight per cent as a reason for stopping breast feeding in the first six weeks, and by 11 per cent between six weeks and four months. Care of the baby can more easily be done, they say, by a friend or relative using a formula bottle feed. Many drugs contraindicate breast feeding, such as anticoagulants, anticonvulsants, antithyroid drugs, narcotics, lithium salts, iodides and bromides, sulfonamides, barbiturates and steroids. The usefulness of formula milk is obvious here.

Other factors must also be considered when assessing why bottle feeding is more popular in the long term than breast feeding. If a mother needs to rest, or to involve other people in caring for her child, it is probably easier and quicker to mix a bottle feed than to express breast milk. The satisfaction of seeing the milk going into the baby, and of knowing how much has been taken, can be psychologically very important. Also to be taken into account is the fact that breast feeding, unlike bottle feeding, has a reputation of being tiring, although this is hard to distinguish from postpartum recovery in many cases.

It is to the credit of the baby formula manufacturers that a high quality formula, broadly approximating to many of the components of average human milk, is available.

References

1. Department of Health and Social Security, 1988. Present Day Practice in Infant Feeding: Third Report. Report on Health and Social Subjects 32. HMSO
2. Department of Health and Social Security, 1974. Present Day Practice in Infant Feeding. Report on Health and Social Subjects 9. HMSO
3. Department of Health and Social Security, 1980. Present Day Practice in Infant Feeding: 1980. Report on Health and Social Subjects 20. HMSO
4. Fomon S J, Filer L J, Anderson T A, Ziegler E E, 1979. Recommendations for Feeding Normal Infants. Paediatrics, 63, 52-59
5. Wharton B A, 1982. Past Achievements and Future Priorities – a view of present day practice in infant feeding 1980. In: Nutrition and Health: a Perspective, ed. Turner M R. MTP Press, London
6. Hooper M and Newell D, 1987. Are Mothers Prepared for Breast Feeding? Maternal and Child Health, 114–117
7. Gillie O, 1988. Report Encourages Women to Breast Feed for One Year. The Times, London
8. Jelliffe D B and Jelliffe E F P, 1978. Human Milk in the Modern World. Oxford Medical Publications, OUP
9. World Health Organisation, 1981. International Code of Marketing of Breast Milk Substitutes. WHO, Geneva
10. Martin J and Monk J, 1982. Infant Feeding 1980. Social Survey Division of OPCS, HMSO
11. Katcher A L and Lanese M G, 1985. Breast Feeding of Employed Mothers: a reasonable accommodation in the workplace. Paediatrics, 75, 644-647
12. Sloper K and Baum J D, 1974. Patterns of Infant Feeding in Oxford. Archives of Disease in Childhood, 49, (9), 749
13. UNICEF, 1988. The State of the World's Children 1988. OUP

CHAPTER 6

Practical physiology and management of breast feeding

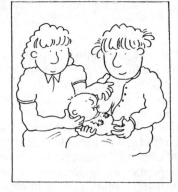

Throughout history the survival of our species has depended mainly on the supply of human milk. Physiologically and anatomically, most human mothers are designed and equipped to suckle their offspring. The presence of the breast in a newborn baby's mouth will encourage the baby to feed, though mother and baby may need to be helped to achieve this.

In theory breast feeding is a natural and manageable function, only going wrong when there is illness or abnormality. In every society it is a process that has to be learned. In less sophisticated societies, where choices and alternatives are not always available and survival depends on success, it is taught by example.

Sophisticated industrial societies present greater social and familial influences, and a completely different set of psychological and behavioural mechanisms exist, so that in practice greater numbers of women do not succeed, many choosing not to breast feed at all.

It is worth noting that a high proportion of women in England and Wales who were successful in breast feeding, were themselves breast fed and were influenced in their choice by their mothers and husbands.[1]

Giving milk is a function of the whole woman, in which her personality and attitudes are involved in conjunction with the complex physical and chemical activities of her body,[2] while the size, vigour and searching abilities of her baby make an important contribution to her ability to breast feed.[3]

Successful breast feeding also appears to be greatly helped by early post partum contact. Gunther suggests that the baby should go to the breast as soon as possible, because early stimulation of the breast is necessary to induce the formation of enough milk in two days' time. It also makes a subsequent abundance of milk more likely.[4,5]

Normal women will experience the same hormonal and physical changes in pregnancy, but they will not all be equally successful at breast feeding. Breast feeding is greatly influenced by infinitely variable emotional and psychological factors, so that no two breast feeding women, nor any two breast fed babies, are alike.

Physiology

There are three stages in the production of milk. First the breasts must become larger to accommodate the milk (mammogenesis). Then milk secretion must be started and a supply of milk created (lactogenesis). Finally the milk supply must be maintained (galactopoiesis).

All these processes result from a complex interaction of a variety of hormones among which prolactin, oestrogens and progesterone are prominent, but the precise way in which these events are brought about is not yet fully understood. It is known that the level of oestrogen begins increasing in the mother a few weeks before her baby is born, and that it increases rapidly during the last two weeks and falls dramatically at birth.

The third stage, the maintenance of the milk supply, depends on the baby's sucking at the breast to stimulate the release of oxytocin by the posterior lobe of the pituitary gland. This causes the cells around the alveoli, as well as the uterus, to contract, and causes the 'let down' (initiation of milk flow) two or three days after parturition.

During the interval between birth and the 'let down', the baby feeds on colostrum, a uniquely protein-rich liquid which the alveolar cells of the breast have been secreting from as early as the fourth month of pregnancy. Colostrum is all the nourishment the newborn infant needs for the first day of life outside the womb, and it eases the transition from placental feeding to milk feeding.

After two or three days, the baby begins to take its mother's milk. Adequately nourished mothers will produce about 600 ml per day in the early stages, increasing to about 750 to 850 ml per day at six months.[4,5] More milk is produced in the morning than in the evening.[6,7]

The 'let down' reflex or draught reflex

The 'let down' reflex, which produces a tingling sensation in the breasts followed by a feeling of fullness, is the term applied to the mechanism which stimulates the flow of milk from the alveoli (the secretory cells) to the lactiferous sinuses (the reservoirs). It is triggered by the baby suckling, and is susceptible to emotional and psychological influences that can effectively stem the flow of milk. It can also be stimulated by extraneous influences. The sight or sound of her baby, or even of another baby, will sometimes cause a breast feeding mother to produce milk. Not all women who breast feed successfully, however, get this sensation of 'let down'.

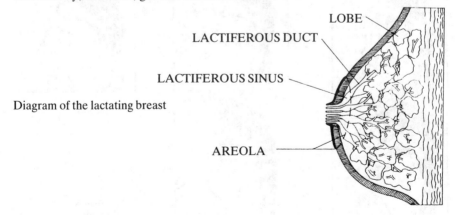

LOBE

LACTIFEROUS DUCT

LACTIFEROUS SINUS

Diagram of the lactating breast

AREOLA

It is necessary to distinguish milk flow from milk secretion, especially when teaching mothers manual expression. Secretion takes place in the breast, influenced by prolactin from the anterior pituitary, and by demand. If no milk is withdrawn, secretion ceases. If the baby is large, or if there are twins, more milk is secreted than if the baby is small, the control of milk from the breast being first nervous then hormonal.

Any stimulation of the nipple and the areola causes the discharge of oxytocin from the posterior pituitary gland which acts on the smooth muscle of the breast, so that it actively expels the milk into the large ducts by causing the cells around the alveoli to contract. Expulsion occurs not only in the stimulated breast, but to some extent in the other breast as well. The contraction around the alveoli is usually felt by the mother, and is sometimes described as 'nearly a pain'. As well as the 'let down', it is sometimes called the 'draught reflex', and occurs 30 to 90 seconds after the first stimulation of the nipple. The quick expulsion of milk may make the baby gulp and choke, after which the baby obtains milk only by steady sucking.

Psychological control of the draught reflex can often be substituted for physical control. For example, the draught reflex may be felt at the usual feeding time even when the mother and baby are apart, while an over-anxious mother may unconsciously suppress it. Mothers should be told that it is normal to have a conditioned reflex when sight or sound of the child will produce a flow of milk, that milk may flow from the breast opposite to the one at which the baby is feeding, and that they may experience abdominal cramps caused by uterine contractions, especially while the uterus is returning to normal.

Breast management

There have been two views about breast management in pregnancy. One view was that during the last three to four months, the duct system of the

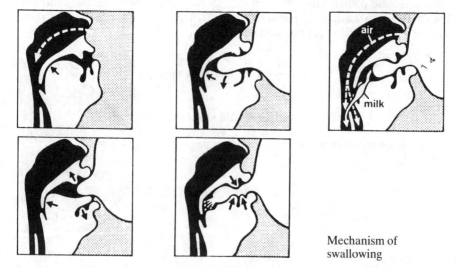

Mechanism of swallowing

breasts should be kept open by regular expression to remove stale colostrum, to keep the nipple sinuses clear, and to improve the milk flow in the puerperium. It was also thought to give mothers experience in handling their breasts, and so perhaps to help some women to overcome their antipathy to breast feeding which expresses itself as a fear of having their breasts touched.

A currently more acceptable view is that women do not need to be encouraged to handle their breasts because the duct system will take care of itself. This does not overcome the problem of the woman who has a genuine fear of having her breasts touched. While it should be emphasised that nothing should be done to interfere with the natural production of colostrum, a gentle and sensitive approach should be taken to the woman who has a real physical antipathy to breast feeding. Making her feel inadequate at this state may inhibit breast feeding later.

In some women colostrum leaks during pregnancy, and breast pads may need to be worn inside the bra, especially towards the end. Other women do not notice the existence of colostrum at all until after the birth. In neither case is there any difference in the production of milk, nor in the success of breast feeding.

How a baby suckles

In suckling, a baby draws the nipple and areola into the posterior oral cavity, and brings the tongue, and the front part of the roof of the mouth, into close approximation to the lactiferous sinuses which lie under the areola. The baby, by pushing the tongue upwards, squeezes the milk out of the lactiferous sinuses, through the small openings in the nipples, into the back of the mouth. The gums are not used during breast feeding, which can continue even when teeth are present.

A 'biting' baby should be told firmly 'No', and is usually just experimenting with new teeth. Though painful and unpleasant at the time, it rarely continues, and breast feeding can be resumed painlessly again!

Hand expression

It is impossible to copy exactly the baby's mechanism of extracting milk from the breast, which is why continued use of hand or pump expression will gradually diminish the milk supply. However, if the mother and baby need to be separated, and continued feeding of breast milk is desired, hand expression can be taught by an experienced helper − ideally a breast feeding counsellor, midwife or health visitor.

The breast should be supported by the hand, and the lactiferous sinuses gently compressed between the ball of the thumb and the palmar surface of the forefinger, which should be kept straight. If the thumb is also directed towards the nipple, this will further assist the flow of the milk out of the sinuses into a sterile receptacle, which can be held by the mother's other hand, or placed on a table conveniently in front of her. Pressure should be exerted at short rhythmic intervals, allowing time for the lactiferous sinuses to refill.

No pressure should be exerted on the breast tissue, as it is not possible to

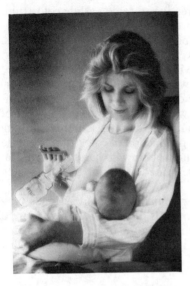

Hand expression can be tiring and some mothers prefer to use a breast-pump. Milk will often flow more easily into the pump if the mother expresses it while feeding her baby on the other breast.

express milk other than by emptying the lactiferous sinuses. 'Nipping' or pinching should be avoided, as it is liable to damage the tissue. However, some women find it helpful to massage the breasts before hand expression, and will need experienced help with this.

Some women, when their breasts are very full and tense, find hand expression helpful in relieving the pressure before the baby is put to the breast. With careful handling and help, however, the baby will do the job satisfactorily, and the fullness will gradually diminish as the milk flow adjusts to the baby's needs.

If the baby is in the special care baby unit and cannot be breast fed, collecting milk by hand expression is an excellent way to ensure that the baby is fed on breast milk, and gives a mother the satisfaction of knowing that she is giving her baby her own milk.

Sore nipples should not make it necessary to express milk by hand. In such a case, the mother needs to be taught how to attach the baby properly to her breast. Unless this is achieved, the problem will recur.

Babies with cleft palate or harelip can also be given breast milk from a spoon, a bottle or a special feeder (see Chapter 10) if the mother is encouraged to express her milk. However, hand expression to empty the breasts completely can be very tiring to the fingers, and the use of a breast pump should be considered. In mild cases, breast feeding may be possible with extra help, and the mother should be encouraged to persevere. After surgery, breast feeding should be re-commenced as soon as possible.

Cleanliness

Mothers should be advised to wash their hands before handling their breasts, and before breast feeding. A clean towel should be kept and used for this purpose alone. Nipples and breasts must be kept clean, but ritual washing before each feed is unnecessary, and may interfere with the natural contact between mother and child.

Breast feeding

It is important for mother and baby to be in a comfortable position.

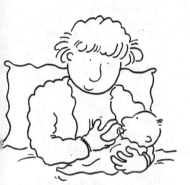

Sitting up in bed, baby's head cradled by the arm. Mother's back must be well supported.

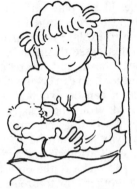

Sitting on chair, back supported, baby on pillow on mother's lap.

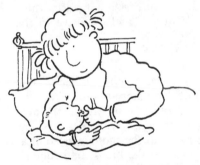

Lying beside baby. Helpful if stitches are sore.

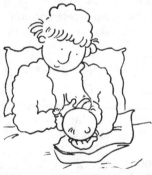

Baby on pillow under mother's arm, feet extended behind her, head supported by mother's hand. Helpful after Caesarean section.

If a baby's cheek is stroked or held against a mother's breast, the baby will turn towards it and seek the nipple, which will contract, enabling the baby to grasp it more easily. This is known as the baby's rooting reflex. The baby's mouth should reach the nipple easily, and the nasal airway must be kept clear.

To prevent sore nipples, it is important to ensure that the baby's mouth takes most of the areola as well as the nipple. When the baby takes the breast it creates a vacuum, which can only be broken by the baby letting go, or by the mother inserting her finger in the side of the baby's mouth. The baby can then be gently removed from the breast. Mothers should be taught how to release the vacuum in this way, and warned that simply pulling the baby off the breast can cause sore nipples.

At first the baby may not require all the milk from both breasts, and may feed contentedly from one side only. The mother will not need reminding which side is due to be emptied!

Some babies like to play with the nipple when they have finished sucking. Mothers should be reassured that this is quite normal, and is part of the baby's instinct to explore its environment. If a baby takes too much milk, it may regurgitate ('possett') the milk: this also is normal. Occasionally a whole feed is vomited back, and the parents should be reassured that this is not unusual. Another feed can be given after a short rest.

Swallowed air can be expelled by holding the baby in a sitting position, leaning forwards from the waist and supported by the mother's arm. The object of this is to bring the cardiac orifice of the stomach in line with the posterior pharynx, so that the baby can 'burp up' the swallowed air. The likelihood of swallowing air is greatly reduced if the mother has learned how to get the baby to suckle at the breast properly.

Teaching a mother how to breast feed should ideally be started during her pregnancy, because when she is newly delivered, she is tired and emotionally vulnerable. Once the baby is born, the mother needs extra support and encouragement, as well as practical help to maintain her confidence in herself as a mother. Casual remarks and ribaldry by the professional staff, which seem harmless and friendly to them, may be hurtful and offensive to the mother.

Feeding immediately after birth

Mothers and babies differ, so there can be no hard and fast rules. Time schedules are often designed to suit the staff of the maternity unit where the baby is born, and if the mother finds that she is out of gear with it, she may abandon breast feeding instead of simply abandoning the schedule. It is now generally accepted that the baby should be given to the mother as soon as possible after the delivery, and putting the baby to the breast immediately after the birth aids the third stage of labour and the involution of the uterus. There is evidence, too, that mothers who nurse and suckle their babies soon after birth are able to start breast feeding earlier than those who wait for a day.[5]

The first few days

During the first few days colostrum is produced. At about the third day, the milk secretion and flow start to be established. Feeding on demand in these early days will enable mother and baby to establish a sequence which is satisfactory to them both. Breast fed babies generally require three-hourly feeding at first, but more frequent feeds are not unusual. A wakeful baby requiring more frequent feeds will not necessarily cause sore nipples.[8,8A] In the early days, a feeding bottle should not be used, as the baby may refuse to acquire the more difficult skill of breast feeding.

Some mothers may like to offer cooled, boiled water on a sterilised spoon between feeds. Extra fluids are not necessary, but can be given as reassurance, especially in hot weather or if the baby has a high temperature.

During the first few days, a baby who remains asleep for more than four hours after a feed, or who is sleepy and difficult to rouse, will need careful observation. Quiet, undemanding babies should not be dismissed as 'good'. Dehydration and weight loss occur quickly if a baby is frequently left for too long between feeds. Premature, very sick or 'small for dates' babies will be especially at risk, and will need to be awakened for regular feeds and observation.

After ten days

As stated earlier, the most frequent reason that mothers give for abandoning breast feeding is a shortage of milk. However, if breast feeding has been started successfully, the milk supply is unlikely to diminish by itself (though it may be affected by factors like anxiety, lack of rest, or inadequate diet). In general, demand creates supply, and unless feeding is stopped, the milk supply should not decline.

Feeding for 'ten minutes a side' is completely outdated.[8A] Some babies suck very rapidly, and may take all they need in five to seven minutes at each breast. Other babies may suckle slowly because the milk is flowing slowly, or because they need pauses to expel swallowed air.

Feeding should be a relaxed affair. The mother should be comfortable and prepared for longish feed times, perhaps as long as one hour at first. She should be given simple tips, such as making sure she has something to drink, seeing to other children's needs before she starts feeding, and leaving the phone off the hook, all of which will contribute to a more relaxed event. Some babies will demand more frequent feeds, and may be more demanding in the latter part of the day, since less milk is produced at this time. If the mother knows that this is normal, she is more likely to accept the situation, and will not feel that she is failing to satisfy her baby. Interestingly enough, bottle fed babies are also often unsettled in the latter part of the day, which indicates that other factors influence behaviour, not just the fact that less milk is available at this time.

Weighing

It is wrong to pay too little or too much attention to baby's weight gains and losses. The mother must not be allowed to remain distressed because her baby fails to gain in one particular week, or when the average gain is steady but smaller than expected. Infants normally lose weight during the first few days after birth, but this is usually regained by the tenth to fourteenth day. During this period, mothers may need reassurance that everything is all right. If a mother's anxiety is unrelieved, she may panic and change to bottle feeding.

The baby who fails to gain weight in two successive weeks, or who loses weight, should be examined medically to exclude all possible causes of failure to thrive. Test weighing should be discouraged in the community, as the scales can be inaccurate and mothers are alarmed unnecessarily. If the baby is at risk, then medical help should be sought.

The amount of milk taken at a feed is so variable that a single test feed is useless, and for recordings to be valid at all they must be made over a 24 hour period. The anxiety caused in that time can be very damaging.

There is normally some variation in the amount of milk taken at each feed. The intake for average sized babies is 150 ml per kilogram of body weight per day (2.5 oz per pound). Small babies may take as much as 220 ml per kg per day (3.5 oz per lb) before gaining weight. Large babies may require relatively less than average, for example 125 ml per kg per day (2 oz per lb).

It is important to realise that breast fed babies may also be underfed due to inadequate intake of breast milk, and it is important to be alert to this possibility and, if possible, to remedy it. If the mother and baby are well, inadequate intake of breast milk is nearly always a management problem, which can be resolved by overseeing the feeds and pin-pointing the problem. It is important to ensure that the mother has enough to eat and drink, and is resting sufficiently in the early weeks.

'Top-up' and 'replacement' feeds

The terms 'supplementary feed' and 'complementary feed' are often used to refer to bottle feeds which are given in addition to, or instead of, breast feeds. Unfortunately, different people use these two terms in exactly opposite ways, and one cannot always be sure which term has which meaning.

We shall therefore use neither of these terms, but shall use the following instead.

A **top-up feed** is one that is given in addition to, and immediately following, a breast feed.

A **replacement feed** is one that is given instead of a breast feed. Note that it may consist of breast milk previously expressed by the mother: the point is that a baby does not take it direct from the mother's breast, but from a bottle or other feeding device.

When breast milk is not used, approved modified cows' milk formulas are used instead. Ante-natal education is important to prevent the wrong milk foods being used, as these are dangerous, and may even be lethal, to a new baby.

Neither top-up nor replacement feeds should be necessary when mother and baby are fit and well. If the baby needs to be separated from the mother, then replacement feeds must be given, if possible consisting of the mother's own milk.

The introduction of top-up feeds, however well intended, often means the gradual cessation of breast feeding. The more top-ups are offered, the less breast milk is produced. The baby becomes dissatisfied, and the top-ups become even more necessary. Gradually the top-up feeds replace the breast feeds.

Replacement feeds may be thought to be helpful when a baby is unsettled after feeding, or when the mother is tired and needs a break from frequent breast feeding. (Top-up feeding may even be suggested here, which will be unhelpful in the long run.) Often the mother feels that her milk is insufficient, and lacks the confidence to rely on her own milk supply.

All these situations can normally be remedied with reassurance and support, especially in the early days. Feeding patterns can be erratic and there may be minor difficulties, all of which are normal and may even be expected while both mother and baby are still recovering from the birth. Well-meaning professionals can do more harm than they realise by suggesting top-up or replacement feeds, especially if the mother is very keen to succeed in breast feeding. A mother's confidence may go when her baby cries at a half empty breast, but settles when given a bottle feed.

However, it is important to know that with perseverance and hard work, it is often possible to re-establish milk production by putting the baby back on the breast regularly. Women who have adopted babies have been known to stimulate milk production in this way, even if they have not given birth.

Top-up feeds should be discouraged and cease as soon as breast milk is well established again, which one may reasonably hope it will be with more frequent feeding.

Weight gain is one obvious sign of a healthy baby. However, unless the baby is small for dates, premature or unwell, a week or two without gain does not necessarily mean that top-up or replacement feeds should be advised. The needs of the individual mother and baby must be assessed. Monitoring should include other indicators of good health besides weight gain.

Is the baby getting enough food?

The following are some guides to whether the baby is getting enough food.

1. Appearance and general behaviour.

2. Weight gain is usually 142 to 225 g (5 to 8 oz) per week for the first three months.[10] Note that some babies have a cycle of weight gain over two to three weeks, e.g. they may gain less weight in one week, but make up the expected gain by two weeks later.

3. Alertness when awake and, after feeds, a short period of tranquillity followed by falling asleep.

4. Warm and silky skin, and firm but elastic subcutaneous tissue.

5. Pink mucous membranes.

6. Abdomen prominent after feeding, but not distended.

7. Urine and stools passed easily, and of normal colour and frequency.

8. Moving and kicking well. Crying lustily for food; crying if cold or insecure, but not having prolonged crying spells.

9. Sleeping well between feeds.

Feeding schedules

Illingworth made the following observations in a study of 237 babies, 131 of whom were on self demand feeding and 106 on a rigid schedule.[11]

1. Many demand babies took frequent feeds from the fourth to the eighth days. On the fifth day 36 (28.6%) took eight feeds or more, and 12 took nine feeds or more.

2. Babies on self demand feeding gained weight more rapidly than those on a rigid schedule.

3. There was a strong correlation between the number of feeds in 24 hours, the amount of milk taken (ascertained by test feeds) and the weight gain.

4. Sore nipples and over-distended breasts occurred twice as often in mothers of babies on a rigid schedule.

5. Babies who were initially on self demand feeding were significantly more often fully breast fed on discharge from hospital, and at one month old.

Some mothers feel happier trying to keep feeds to a schedule of 3 to 4 hours, and it is not good practice to recommend that a breast feeding mother should cut out the night feeds. However, a healthy breast fed baby that sleeps through the night should be left to do so.

Premature, small for dates and unwell babies may need more frequent feeds both night and day, to increase their weight.

For specific medical reasons, a mother may be asked to feed her baby at regular intervals, waking if necessary, until the health and weight of her baby are satisfactory.

The mother's well-being

An adequate and well balanced diet is important for the breast feeding mother. Her daily intake should consist of a good mixed diet containing some dairy products, meats (or protein equivalents, e.g. lentils, other pulses or nuts), cereal foods and plenty of fresh fruits and vegetables.

Isolated mothers in particular need encouragement to get out and about. Plenty of exercise and fresh air is important, as well as the social contacts made outside the home. In the early weeks, rest periods are vital, since over tiredness and anxiety can lead to depression. Help in the home, and some free time to relax and socialise, are the ideal. Emphasis should be placed on the role of the father, and the mother should be encouraged to find time to relax with him. At the same time the father should be encouraged to support her, and to give time to learning how to cope with the needs of the new baby.

The mother's emotional well-being is as important to feeding her baby as her physical well-being. A tense, anxious, unhappy mother is less likely to continue with the commitment of breast feeding, and will more easily give up when problems arise.

Some problems of breast feeding

Some problems can be anticipated during the ante-natal period, and advice should be given. Anxieties can be discussed and allayed. Preparation for breast feeding starts with good education.

Retracted nipples may be helped with the use of nipple shells. While it is thought that the baby has the best 'method' of solving this problem, by suckling, the mother will need help in getting the baby to take the breast initially.

All the conditions listed below can normally be overcome with careful management and treatment: but if the mother finds the condition so painful that she wants to abandon breast feeding, her wishes should be respected. The object is not to go to war with the mother, but to feed the baby.

Sore nipples occur if the baby is not applied properly to the breast during feeding.

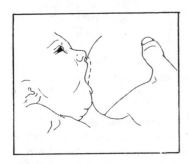 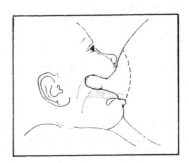

Correct position of tongue
in relation to nipple and gums.
Many mothers need to be taught
to attach their babies properly.

A soft rubber nipple shield (see picture) may give temporary relief from a sore nipple, but it should be used with caution. Continuous use will inhibit the proper sucking response, and hence ultimately milk production.[8] If the mother keeps getting sore nipples, the baby is not taking the breast properly, and mother and baby will need help to achieve this.

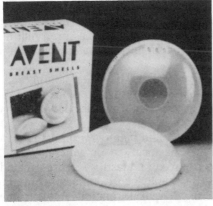 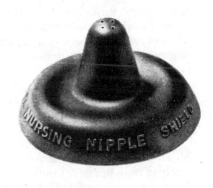

Breast shells   Nipple shield

Babies who are given bottle feeds, especially early on, may find it difficult to get used to the different shape of the nipple. The bottle teat is easier to grip, and the mechanisms of sucking are different. Thus a baby who 'bottle feeds' at the breast will give rise to sore nipples very quickly (see pictures).

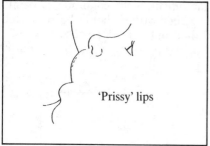

'Prissy' lips

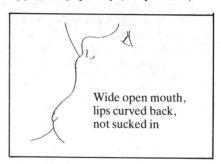

Wide open mouth, lips curved back, not sucked in

Baby 'bottle-feeding' at the breast

Baby sucking correctly at the breast

Breast engorgement is a painful accumulation of secreted milk in the breast which usually occurs on the third or fourth day of lactation. Real engorgement is more than the expected fullness of the breast as the milk comes in, and may occur when the baby's requirements are less than the amount of milk produced. The milk flow mechanism is not functioning properly at this early stage, and if the secretion becomes greater than the amount taken by the baby, milk accumulates and the breasts become distended. If this becomes excessive, the pressure within the breast compresses the veins and the lymphatics draining the breast, and oedema starts to form. The secretion must be removed, otherwise the distension worsens, the pain becomes intense, and the baby cannot suckle. Engorgement may be prevented, at least partly, by getting the baby to feed as soon as possible after birth and by feeding on demand.

In treating engorgement, the breasts must be emptied, and the baby is the best 'device' for doing this. Milk may need to be expressed after feeds, by hand or by pump, during the first few days after milk comes into the breast.

Analgesics may be required, and the mother should be reassured that the engorgement will pass in two or three days. A supportive bra may be helpful to some women.

It is desirable not to refer to breast engorgement, and other painful breast conditions, merely as a 'discomfort'. This is a term often favoured by professionals, possibly in the hope that a euphemism will cause the pain to go away!

Mastitis: The breasts can become inflamed and painful without the presence of infection, and the condition may be localised or general, though rarely in both breasts at once. Infection can result if mastitis is left untreated. The commonest cause of infective mastitis is staphylococcal infection entering through cracked or broken skin, leading to pus formation and eventual discharge through the nipple. Dirty hands and stale milk will cause the problem or perpetuate it. Treatment is with the appropriate antibiotics, to prevent abscess formation.

Acute intramammary mastitis: Lobules in the breast become full of stale milk if not emptied adequately. The distension causes pressure and the formation of a lump which can be felt on examination. There is pain, tenderness and a red flush over the affected area. The mother may have flu-like symptoms and a raised temperature.

Again, treatment begins by emptying the breast, preferably by getting the baby to feed adequately. Massage and warm compresses may help to disperse the lump. Surprisingly, not all cases are infected despite the 'ill' state of the mother.[12] However, untreated mastitis is the principal cause of breast abscess.

Breast feeding should be encouraged to continue, whether there is infection or not. Antibiotics may cause some harmless intermittent diarrhoea in the baby, and both mother and baby may be more susceptible to *candida albicans* (thrush) infection.

Breast abscess: If intramammary mastitis is not successfully treated by emptying and/or by antibiotics, staphylococcal infection (if it arises) may lead to abscess formation. Antibiotic treatment may still stop the infection, preventing the need for surgical incision and drainage. The baby should feed from the unaffected side, and milk from the affected side should be expressed, and discarded if there is pus. Normal breast feeding should be resumed as soon as possible.

Infection of Montgomery tubercles: These structures are near the areola and are superficial. Breast feeding can continue while local treatment to the area of inflammation is given.

Milk leakage: While breast feeding, most women leak some milk from the breast which is not being suckled. This leakage lasts a few moments, and the amount varies from woman to woman. Leaking between feeds occurs when the 'let down' reflex is stimulated. Many women need to wear breast pads in their bras for several months to prevent embarrassing leaks into their clothes.

Poor sucking: Among causes of poor sucking may be the following.

1. An unsettled baby may be communicating some very obvious discomfort such as a dirty nappy, uncomfortable clothes, being over-dressed in a heated room, or having cold extremities. Every baby is an individual, and minor discomforts become important to one and not to another. For example, some babies will happily feed with a dirty nappy, while others will refuse.

2. An ill baby.

3. An aggressive, irritable baby who may be reacting to a nervous or insecure mother. Reassure the mother that there is no abnormality, and that she is the best person to calm her baby. Warn her that nothing is achieved by trying to force a fighting baby. Advise her to take the baby from the breast, settle it, and start again.

4. A sleepy baby. This is not a cause for concern, provided that there is no abnormality and that weight gain is satisfactory. The baby can be taken off

the breast after a reasonable suckling period, and tried again after some stimulation. The mother should be advised not to worry, and to give more frequent feeds for shorter periods. Babies with jaundice, or following a difficult birth, may remain sleepy for a few days, and may need to be wakened for feeds.

Over-feeding: This is very rare in breast feeding, although excessive weight gains do occasionally occur. The baby will usually regurgitate any excess milk.

Weaning from breast to bottle feeds

Weaning from the breast should always be a gradual process, to prevent engorgement. If a mother is able to breast feed for only a few weeks, and has to wean onto a bottle fairly quickly, this can be done over a ten day period by omitting one additional breast feed every alternate day. It does not really matter in which sequence the feeds are changed, and the following regime is given for guidance only.

From day 1: omit 10 a.m. breast feed and substitute a bottle feed.

From day 3: omit   6 p.m. breast feed and substitute a bottle feed.

From day 5: omit   2 p.m. breast feed and substitute a bottle feed.

From day 7: omit 10 p.m. breast feed and substitute a bottle feed.

From day 9: omit   6 a.m. breast feed and substitute a bottle feed.

Where no haste is necessary, weaning can be spread over three months.

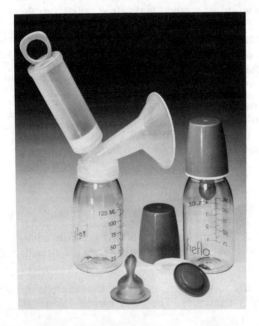

Hand-operated breast pump.
The pump reservoir also
acts as a feeding bottle.

Breast pumps

Breast pumps can be used for the same purposes as hand expression and, in addition, are useful for pulling out slightly retracted or flat nipples immediately before putting the baby to the breast, and for relieving a distended breast before feeding starts. All breast pumps must be sterilised before use, as must any containers used for collecting the milk.

References

1. Martin J, 1976. Infant Feeding 1975. Attitudes and practice in England and Wales. HMSO
2. Newton N, 1971. Psychologic differences between breast and bottle feeding. American Journal of Clinical Nutrition, 24, 993.
3. Jelliffe D B and Jelliffe E F P, 1977. Human Milk in the Modern World. OUP
4. Gunther M, 1976. The New Mother's View of Herself. In: Breast Feeding and the Mother. CIBA Symposium 1976. CIBA Foundation, London
5. Sosa R et al, 1976. The Effect of Early Mother-Infant Contact on Breast Feeding, Infection and Growth. In: Breast Feeding and the Mother. CIBA Symposium 1976, 45. CIBA Foundation, London
6. Lonnderdal B, Forsum E and Hambraeus L, 1976. The Protein Content of Human Milk 11: a longitudinal study of normal material. In: Food and Immunology, 12. Swedish Nutritional Foundation, Stockholm
7. Jelliffe E F P, 1976. Maternal Nutrition and Lactation. In: Breast Feeding and the Mother. CIBA Symposium 1976, 45 (New Series). CIBA Foundation, London
8. Marsh G N, 1985. Modern Obstetrics in General Practice. OUP
8A. Royal College of Midwives 1988. Successful Breast Feeding – practical guide for midwives. Publ. Holywell Press, Oxford
9. Derek Llewellyn Jones, 1983. Breast Feeding: How to Succeed. Publ. Faber & Faber
10. Jolly H, 1985. Book of Child Care. Publ. George Allen & Unwin
11. Illingworth R S and Stone D G H, 1952. Self-demand Feeding in a Maternity Unit. Lancet, 1, 6, 8, 3
12. Gunther M, 1970. Infant Feeding. Publ. Methuen

CHAPTER 7

Bottle feeding

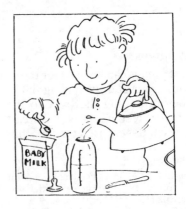

Introduction

Despite the important advantages of breast feeding and its active promotion by health professionals, most mothers choose to bottle feed their babies for a greater part of the first six months.

The milk of each mammalian species differs in its composition, and is highly adapted to meet the specific nutritional and physiological needs of the newborn animal for which it is intended. Historically, the wide availability of cows' milk has meant that infants who were not breast fed were given cows' milk in one form or another as a substitute.

However, the nutritional requirements of the young calf are very different from those of a human baby, and this is reflected in the many significant differences in the milk of the two species (Table 3.2). Due to its high levels of protein and minerals (especially sodium and phosphorus), and its low lactose content, cows' milk needs to be substantially modified before it is fed to infants. This modification is an important aspect of the manufacture of infant formulas, and modern products have nutrient levels which in many respects closely resemble breast milk.

Another important factor is the availability of nutrients for absorption in the immature gut. Young babies are prone to malabsorb certain types of nutrients, e.g. saturated fats; and the nutrients in breast milk may, in any case, be better absorbed than those in infant formulas, e.g. iron. Thus the absorption factor needs to be borne in mind when making a comparison between the levels of nutrients in the two feeds. In addition, at the present time infant formulas contain none of the anti-infective components which are present in breast milk.

In recent years the composition of infant formulas has improved considerably. These changes were introduced in response to far-reaching recommendations made by the DHSS Panel on Child Nutrition in 1974.[1] The Panel found that certain clinical problems occasionally seen in bottle fed infants were a direct result of inappropriately high levels of protein, sodium and phosphorus in the formulas used at that time.

This situation was exacerbated by parents adding extra scoops of powder, or compressing powder into the scoops, which resulted in feeds containing even higher levels of these nutrients. Problems found at that time included hyperosmolar dehydration, neonatal tetany and obesity. These have now been largely eradicated following the widespread introduction in the middle and late 1970's of low electrolyte formulas and better health education.

Detailed compositional guidelines for infant formulas have been published by the DHSS[2] and all present-day products conform to these standards. An EEC directive will ultimately be incorporated into UK law.

Types of infant formula

The main adjustments made to cows' milk in producing a food suitable for infants may include any or all of the following:

1. An increase in the level of carbohydrate to approximately 7 to 9 per cent by the addition of lactose, or a combination of lactose and maltodextrin and, in one formula, starch (amylose).

2. Partial or total replacement of milk fat by vegetable oils, or a mixture of vegetable oils and animal fat, to improve the absorption characteristics in the intestine.

3. Reduction of the protein content to between 1.5 and 2.0 per cent, and modification of the ratio of insoluble casein to soluble whey from 80 : 20 (as in cows' milk) to 40 : 60, the ratio found in mature breast milk.

4. A reduced mineral content, achieved by the dilution effect of adding lactose (or other carbohydrate), or by electrodialysis of the whey protein fraction. This latter process involves the removal of minerals by passing an electric current through liquid whey.

5. The addition of a comprehensive range of minerals and vitamins to provide a nutritionally complete feed.

Infant formulas may conveniently be classified into two groups: first, products containing a casein-to-whey ratio of 40 : 60, known as the **whey dominant** formulas; and second, those which have a casein-to-whey ratio of 80 : 20, known as the **casein dominant** formulas. Compositional details of the whey dominant and casein dominant formulas currently available are shown in Table 7.1, along with corresponding values for the DHSS guidelines.

Theoretically, whey dominant formulas are preferable for younger babies since the amino acid content of the protein is closer to that in mature breast milk, and the levels of sodium, phosphorus and other minerals are lower than those of casein dominant formulas. In practice, however, babies thrive on both types of product, and no important differences have yet been demonstrated between the biological values of the protein in whey dominant and casein dominant formulas.[3]

An interesting question is why there should be two types of infant formula if one is theoretically superior to the other. For reasons that are not clear, particular brands or types of formula do not appear to suit individual babies. Whether this is an imagined phenomenon or a real one is debatable. However, in practice difficulties such as mild vomiting, undue possetting, constipation and lack of satisfaction cause many mothers to change formulas.

In one study of over 4,000 bottle feeding mothers, 44 per cent had changed formulas by the time the baby was 6 to 10 weeks old, and a minority had changed the formula more than once by this age.[3] The most frequent change

TABLE 7.1 Composition of infant formulas compared with DHSS guidelines (1980, 1988)
Values per 100ml

	Energy kJ	kcal	Protein g	Fat g	Carbo-[1] hydrate g	Sodium mg	Potas-sium mg	Calcium mg	Phos-phorus mg	Iron mg	Zinc mg	Vitamin A µg	Vitamin D µg	Vitamin C mg
Whey dominant														
Cow & Gate Premium	275	66	1.5	3.6	7.3	18	65	54	27	0.5	0.4	80	1.1	8
Farley Ostermilk	284	68	1.45	3.82	7.4	19	57	35	29	0.65	0.34	100	1.0	6.9
Milupa Aptamil	281	67	1.5	3.6	7.7	18	85	59	35	0.7	0.4	61	1.0	6
Wyeth SMA Gold Cap	274	65	1.5	3.6	7.2	15	56	42	28	0.67	0.5	79	1.05	5.8
Casein dominant														
Cow & Gate Plus	275	66	1.9	3.4	7.3	25	100	85	55	0.5	0.4	80	1.1	8
Farley Ostermilk 2	273	65	1.7	2.6	9.3	25	86	61	49	0.65	0.33	97	1.0	6.4
Milupa Milumil	290	69	1.9	3.1	8.8	24	85	71	55	0.43	0.41	57	1.0	7.6
Wyeth SMA White Cap	274	65	1.5	3.6	7.2	18	62	46	36	0.67	0.5	79	1.05	5.8
DHSS Guidelines	270– 315	65– 75	1.2– 2.0[2] 1.5– 2.0[3]	2.3– 5.0	4.8– 10.0	15– 35	50– 100	30– 120	15– 60	0.07– 0.7	0.2– 0.64[4]	40– 150	0.7– 1.3	3– ns

[1]Carbohydrate expressed as monosaccharide
[2]Whey dominant formulas
[3]Casein dominant formulas
[4]Tentative guideline

was from a whey dominant formula to a casein dominant formula, and by far the commonest reason given for this change was that the baby was still hungry or not satisfied after feeds.

There is no scientific evidence to demonstrate that casein dominant formulas are more satisfying than whey dominant formulas, and one small scale study which investigated this characteristic failed to show any benefit.[4] If this 'satisfying' effect of casein dominant formulas is real, however, one possible explanation is that casein forms a firm clot in the acidic conditions of the stomach, and its passage through the intestine is slower than that of whey, which remains soluble under these conditions.[2,5] The casein clot might be responsible for a more satisfied baby.

Another interesting fact is that the levels of protein and fat in milk vary according to the mammalian species. Thus the milk of those animals whose feeds are separated by long intervals, e.g. deer, contain more protein and fat than the milk of species that feed more frequently, e.g. goats and humans.[6,7]

Until more evidence is available from research, it is not possible to provide a scientific basis for using casein dominant formulas in preference to whey dominant formulas. Meanwhile, the advice published by the DHSS Working Group[3] appears to be a practical guideline:

> Evidence that hungry infants may be more satisfied by casein dominant than by whey dominant formulas is anecdotal. No harm is likely to result from changing from one to the other and this course, if apparently effective in individual cases, is preferable to the premature introduction of solids.

> In general, however, changing from one formula to another, as a means of combating some ill-defined problem, is not recommended until other possible causes have been ruled out. A very small percentage of babies require special formulas, e.g. soya based, hydrolysed protein etc. They should be under the direct care of a doctor, and ideally the parents should receive practical support from a dietitian.

Soya formulas

During recent years, several soya based formulas have become widely available and their use, although small at the present time, is slowly growing. These products are free from cows' milk and ingredients derived from it, such as lactose, and they are primarily intended for infants who are allergic to cows' milk or who have a lactose intolerance.

They may also be used for managing certain rare inherited disorders of metabolism (galactosaemia). Infants who may need to be changed onto a soya formula should first be referred to their general practitioner for a diagnosis. Once the doctor is satisfied that a soya formula is necessary, one of the following approved products may be prescribed:

Formula S	(Cow & Gate)
Wysoy (contains beef fat)	(Wyeth)
Prosobee	(Mead Johnson)
Isomil	(Abbott Laboratories)
Ostersoy	(Farley Health Products)

It is important to note that other soya milks, goats' milk and ewes' milk, which are available in health food shops and supermarkets, are not nutritionally complete or balanced, and are not suitable for feeding to infants.[2,3,9]

Quantity of milk

The needs of individual babies vary considerably. As a general rule, however, the quantity of milk a baby will consume is approximately 150ml per kilogram of body weight per day (2.5 oz per lb per day). This amount of correctly prepared formula (or breast milk) will provide all the infant's requirements of nutrients, energy (Calories) and fluid.

Instruction on bottle feeding

It is the responsibility of health professionals to ensure that all parents, including those who breast feed, fully understand the correct procedure for preparing bottle feeds. The omission of this instruction during ante-natal classes, in the misguided belief that parents will be more likely to breast feed, is irresponsible and could result in a seriously sick baby.

The importance of good hygiene, and care with measuring the water and baby milk powder, need to be clearly explained to parents without causing them undue anxiety. Methods of sterilisation should be discussed and demonstrated, and all parents should be shown how to prepare a feed and be encouraged to practise this themselves.

Preparing the feed

Hands should always be washed before preparing a feed, and the feeding bottles, caps, teats and levelling knife (also mixing spoon and jug if used) should be sterilised either chemically or by boiling.

With the chemical method a sterilising solution recommended for infant feeding equipment is used, and the levelling knife and mixing spoon must be made of plastic, not metal. All the utensils should be submerged for at least the time recommended by the steriliser manufacturer, and they should remain immersed until immediately before the next feed. They must then be rinsed with cooled, freshly boiled water before use.

Alternatively, the equipment should be fully immersed and boiled for three minutes, after which the bottles should be capped until used. Domestic microwave ovens are not effective for sterilising feeding equipment.[10]

Wide-necked simple cylindrical shaped bottles are recommended, since they are easier to clean than bottles with a complex shape.[3] The teat should have an opening of sufficient size to allow the milk to drip slowly through when the bottle is held upside down. The opening should be larger for weak babies, and smaller for vigorously feeding infants.

The mixing instructions given on the milk pack should be carefully adhered to. In the past, milk feeds were often wrongly mixed and became too concentrated. It is therefore important that the mother knows how to use the measuring scoop properly, and she should be taught:

1. To use only the scoop provided with the packet of milk powder being used. Milk powders prepared by different processes have different densities, and therefore scoops are **not** interchangeable between different dried milks.

2. To allow the powder to fill the scoop without applying any pressure.

3. To follow the manufacturer's instructions exactly when mixing milk powder with water, and never to add extra scoops or give fewer scoops.

4. To use the scoop only for measuring the milk powder, and never to use it for measuring water.

The water used for making up feeds must be boiled and cooled to the temperature recommended in the mixing instructions on the baby milk pack.

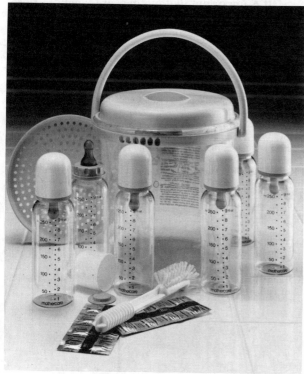

A modern sterilising unit

73

Domestically softened water, or water which has been boiled repeatedly, should not be used, since these will contain higher levels of minerals. Bottled waters are not recommended for preparing infant feeds in the UK, since some contain unacceptably high levels of minerals. In any case, they provide no advantage, since they must be boiled before use.

Feeds may be given at ambient temperature. The temperature of warmed feeds should first be checked by running a few drops onto the inside of the wrist. Infant feeds should not be warmed in a microwave oven once they are in feeding bottles, since fluid at the centre of the bottle may become very hot and could scald the baby.[11]

When more than one bottle is being prepared, sufficient milk powder for the total number of feeds can be mixed in a sterilised jug, and may be stored in individual bottles in a refrigerator for up to 24 hours. Individual bottles can then be warmed immediately before use. Warm feeds should never be stored in a vacuum flask, since micro-organisms thrive under these conditions and could cause gastroenteritis.

After the feed has been given, the bottle and teat should be rinsed thoroughly in cold water, using a bottle brush to remove milk residues. They should then be washed in hot water, using the brush and washing-up liquid to remove fat deposits. Any remaining deposits on the teat may be removed by turning it inside out and scouring with a little salt, though some authorities do not recommend this practice. It is important that mothers are taught to rinse the teat thoroughly afterwards, to remove all traces of salt. The teat and bottle should then be sterilised ready for the next feed.

References

1. Department of Health and Social Security, 1974. Present Day Practice in Infant Feeding. London, HMSO
2. Department of Health and Social Security, 1980. Artificial Feeds for the Young Infant. London, HMSO
3. Department of Health and Social Security, 1988. Present Day Practice in Infant Feeding. Third Report. London, HMSO
4. Brooke C G and Wood C, 1985. Archives of Disease in Childhood, **60**, 577
5. Platt B S, 1961. Federal Proceedings, Suppl 7, 188
6. Klaus M, Dowling S and Kennell J, 1981. Feeding and Behaviour: Three Recent Observations. In: Infant and Child Feeding, ed. Bond T et al. Academic Press, London
7. Widdowson E M, 1984. Lactation and Feeding Patterns in Different Species. In: Health Hazards of Milk. Publ. Bailliere Tindall
8. Taitz L S, 1982. Soy Feeding in Infancy. Archives of Disease in Childhood, **57**, 814–815
9. Tripp J H, Francis D E M, Knight J A and Harries J T, 1979. Infant Feeding Practices: a Cause for Concern. British Medical Journal, **2**, 707–709
10. Biela A and McGill A E J, 1985. Can Baby Feeding Equipment be Sterilised in the Domestic Microwave Oven? Journal of the Royal Society of Health, **4**, 131–132
11. Sando W C, Gallagher K J and Rodgers B M, 1984. Risk Factors for Microwave Scald Injuries in Infants. Journal of Pediatrics, **105**, 864–866

CHAPTER 8

Principles and teaching of mixed feeding

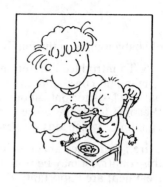

For the first four to six months, breast milk or infant formula and water provide infants with all their nutritional requirements, and the feeding of solid foods before this age is not necessary. The DHSS (1988) advise that infants need a mixed diet when their nutritional requirements are no longer satisfied by milk alone, when their feeding behaviour has progressed from sucking to biting and chewing, and when they are ready to experiment with flavours, textures and consistency.

Surveys (cited[1]) have shown that the first foods usually offered are cereals, rusks and commercial baby foods. There is much to commend pureed and sieved cooked fruits and vegetables, but without the addition of salt or sugar.

Delaying the introduction of solids beyond six months is not to be recommended, since there appears to be a critical age range during which the infant evolves from a sucking to a chewing individual. Some babies have problems accepting varied textures when weaning is delayed, refusing lumpy foods and accepting only purees. In addition, a baby's nutritional requirements at six months are not met by milk alone. Growth rate is probably better than age as an indicator of when to introduce mixed feeding, since each baby is different. Do not be afraid to encourage experimentation and flexibility.

Objects of weaning

The word weaning comes from an Old English word *wenian*, meaning 'to accustom'. The main objects of weaning are:

1. To make the infant less dependent nutritionally on milk. By the age of one year, however, milk should still be an important food, and should desirably provide about 40 per cent of the calorie intake. In real terms, this means about one pint of milk a day, taken as a drink and in cooked dishes.

2. To provide a variety of textures, using pureed and finely diced foods, which will enable the baby ultimately to partake in family meals.

3. To establish the acceptance of a variety of foods having a wide range of flavours.

4. To train the baby to feed with a spoon and to take liquid from a cup. The transformation from breast or bottle feeding to family meals is normally slow, and takes several months to complete. Individual babies vary considerably in their rate of physical and mental development, and these greatly affect the time-scale of the weaning programme. An ideal aim is to have a healthy year-

old baby joining in the family meals, but without added salt and sugar.

5. To introduce different nutrients into the diet, and more iron, since both human and cows' milk are poor sources. A baby has a store of iron at birth but this lasts for only about four to six months, according to his body weight. Weaning foods therefore need to include those which are rich in iron and in vitamin C, which aids the absorption of iron.

Iron deficiency anaemia in toddlers is common[11] and, in Asian children in this country, it may be combined with vitamin D deficiency.[12] Prevention and treatment are important, not only for the well-being of the child but because it is believed that iron deficiency has severe effects on learning, weight gain and psychomotor development.[11,13]

Studies (cited[14]) suggest that infants who are given cows' milk after the age of six months, are more likely to develop iron deficiency if attention is not paid to the iron content of other foods. To avoid this, Tunnessen et al recommend an infant formula which is fortified with iron to be given from 6 to 12 months, or iron supplements. However, it is important not to become over-zealous with iron, as over-supplementation can lead to excess iron storage and susceptibility to infection.

The availability of iron from infant foods is known to be capricious, and depends on the nature and composition of the food. The International Nutrition and Anaemia Consultative Group (cited[15]) suggest that infant weaning foods should be fortified with iron and vitamin C, especially when these are based on soya or cereal, as they are in many developing countries.

Possible indicators for the assessment of iron status are: babies coming from underprivileged homes; babies of Asian families; babies who are introduced early to cows' milk, because not only is this low in iron, but it may induce loss of blood cells from the intestine (cited[14]); and babies who are not receiving iron-fortified cereals, iron-rich weaning foods, iron-fortified milk formula or vitamin C in any form.

Dietary sources of iron

Traditionally, red meat and liver have been considered as the best available sources of iron, and the most readily absorbed. However, as a result of the recommendations of the COMA report,[16] there has been a reduction in the consumption of red meats, which have a higher fat content than white meats, and parents are beginning to ask for information about alternative sources of iron for their babies. Cereals, pulses, bread, cocoa, chocolate drinks and eggs contain iron, but it is poorly absorbed.

While iron from meat is easily absorbed, iron from other foods is better absorbed if vitamin C is given at the same time, as in a drink of blackcurrant or orange juice. Fruits and vegetables contain little iron, but their Vitamin C content performs a useful role by enhancing the availability of iron from non-meat sources. Vegetarian and vegan infants are especially at risk from iron deficiency, and iron fortified foods, including infant formula or follow-up milk, should be recommended.

It is possible that iron absorption may be inhibited if foods are given close to a breast feed (cited[1]), and it may be better to advise that the iron rich foods are given separately.

Introducing solid foods

The introduction of solid foods is often an anxious time for a mother, particularly if the baby is her first. She may need frequent reassurance that her baby is normal and is making satisfactory progress.

It is thought that the early introduction of energy-dense foods may increase the risk of obesity, and may contribute to some chronic allergic illnesses. In addition, solid foods are apt to contain a relatively high renal solute load (sodium, potassium, chloride and protein), which put a stress on the young kidney, particularly if salt is used during cooking or as a condiment.[1]

On the question of obesity, opinion is divided. Harber *et al* found no evidence of obesity associated with the age at which solids were introduced.[2] Wilkinson and Davies, who made a study of fifty primiparae, found that the age of weaning had no influence on growth in the first six months.[3] This was subsequently supported by Barrie, who remarked that babies who were breast fed frequently could become just as fat as those who were bottle fed frequently, and said that the 'early introduction of low-carbohydrate solids is both rational and nutritionally correct.'[4]

There is convincing evidence that early introduction of solids *per se* is not associated with an increased risk of obesity.[5] It depends on the calorie content of the foods being given, and it may be relevant at this stage to indicate the characteristics found in babies who are likely to become fat.

Both parents may be overweight;

Birth weight may be high;

Babies may be finicky;

Babies may have a vigorous feeding style, and have large but less frequent feeds;[6]

They may be less active when awake.[7]

Children who are fat at one year old, and then show a rapid growth in body fat at the age of five to six years, are more likely to remain fat.

Growth charts giving heights and weights for children are helpful[8] though the experienced Health Visitor can usually tell, from an examination of the undressed baby, whether or not there are tell-tale rolls of fat around the trunk, arms or legs. Even so, the factors which influence the development of obesity in childhood are still unclear,[9] though it is a matter for common observation and from longitudinal studies[9] that the prevalence of obesity in children has increased over the past 30 to 40 years, in association with changes in infant feeding habits and general lifestyles. It has been wisely pointed out, however, that in an attempt to reverse these changes, we should not produce a swing towards under-nutrition of babies and children, nor a nation of over-anxious mothers.[10]

The nutritional content of early weaning foods is less important than the acceptance of different flavours and textures. Weaning can be helped if the baby is not too tired or ravenous. Early attempts should be made when other members of the family are not demanding attention. The morning or early afternoon feeds are usually considered to be the best for introducing new foods. A thirsty baby may take the spoon better after a small drink from the breast or bottle, to make him more comfortable and cooperative.

Initially, half to one teaspoon of food should be offered before the normal milk feed. The next day, a little more of the same food is given. After two or three days, when the baby has become used to the new flavour and consistency, another food should be tried.

There is no evidence that offering solid foods at night helps to give a good night's sleep. Indeed, experience shows that it may even keep a baby awake if he is not used to new foods.

Many babies take a dislike to some foods. When this occurs, another food should be given, and the rejected food tried again a few days later. Mealtime battles should be avoided, since they may result in a long-term feeding problem, and an impaired mother-child relationship.

It is worth noting here that although acceptance of different foods by infants during weaning is affected by many factors other than flavour, a study from Minnesota showed that with gentle perseverance over a period of time, most of the infants observed ate a variety of vegetables.[17] The widely-held notion that infants will not eat strong-flavoured vegetables was not supported.

Allergy and food reactions

Babies who have a strong family history of allergy, and especially if one or both parents are atopic, should avoid potentially allergenic foods until they are six months or older. Such foods include cows' milk and cows' milk products (cheese, yogurt etc.), eggs and some fruits, such as strawberries and tomatoes.[10] It may also be wise to avoid wheat, nuts and citrus fruits until the child is older.

Many children 'grow out of' reactions to food by the time they are three years old. The connection between food colourings and preservatives such as tartrazine and benzoic acid, and asthma, eczema and/or urticaria is not clear, but it would seem sensible to avoid foods containing these additives.[19]

Breast fed babies may be sensitised to antigens *via* breast milk. Once the mother's diet is modified to exclude the offending foods, the baby's symptoms may disappear (cited[20]). If dietary restriction is being considered, for either mother or baby, a dietitian's advice is essential.[1] Self-diagnosis of food allergy, and over-restriction of foods offered at weaning, can result in nutritional inadequacies.[21] Similar problems can occur if there is over-zealous application of nutritional guidelines.[16,22] Some ethnic groups tend to delay weaning and allow the child to remain almost exclusively on milk until he is two to three years old. Advisers need to approach this type of problem with extreme tact in order to resolve it.

First foods

Baby cereals are frequently chosen as the first food, since they are easy to prepare, are readily accepted by most infants when mixed with milk, and are economical. Unfortunately, babies find cereals so palatable that mothers may be tempted to feed excessive quantities. Since cereal foods are high in energy (calories), babies can become overweight, and therefore not more than one portion per day should be given.

When cereals are used as a first food, rice-based gluten-free cereals (free from wheat, rye, oats and barley) are often recommended by health professionals. However, many babies dislike baby rice alone and find it more palatable mixed with pureed fruit, such as pear or banana.

Mashed vegetables, such as potatoes or carrots mixed with milk, or mashed banana or finely sieved chicken broth, are all suitable first foods. Egg yolk is frequently recommended for young babies, since it is thought to be a good source of iron. However, the value of this is questionable, since phosphates in the yolk and cooked yolk appear to inhibit iron absorption (cited[23]). When egg yolk is given, it should be cooked until it is firm and then mashed up, perhaps with a little milk from the feed, to soften it. Egg white is not recommended before six months, because some infants may be sensitive to the protein fraction of the albumen.[1]

The commonly held view that gluten-containing foods should be avoided before six months of age is derived from the 1974 DHSS report, *Present Day Practice in Infant Feeding*, which drew attention to the then increasing incidence of coeliac disease and the associated early use of gluten-containing cereals, i.e. before one or two months of age. Since that time, the incidence of coeliac disease has fallen dramatically during infancy, but the reason for this is not clear.

Changes in the diet that have occurred include the later introduction of weaning foods, greater use of gluten-free foods, increased breast feeding and the development of infant formulas which resemble breast milk more closely. As the decline in coeliac disease started before these dietary changes became widespread, other factors such as infection could be involved.[22a] The 1988 DHSS report[1] does not distinguish between gluten-containing and gluten-free foods with respect to age, and recommends their use from about four months.

Salt should never be added to foods for infants. In order to avoid encouraging a taste for sweet foods, and the possible start of dental decay, sugar should not be added to fruit purees and desserts. Milk may be added to stewed fruit, to reduce the sharp flavour of the acids present.

Proprietary weaning foods

Using basic, fresh foods to make up a baby's weaning food is not always easy or convenient, especially when only very small amounts are needed.

This is when proprietary baby foods come into their own. Jars, tins and packets are available in a wide variety of flavours and textures. On the whole they tend to be free from salt, colourings and preservatives, but it is as well to check the list of ingredients carefully since some contain 'hidden' sugars. These 'convenience foods' for a baby should be viewed in the same context as other convenience foods – they are useful on occasions but should not form the baby's total diet.

Introducing cows' milk

As the intake of solid foods increases, the volume of milk offered should gradually be reduced, so that by about the fifth week of weaning, one of the milk feeds can be completely replaced by solids. For the first six months of weaning, breast milk or cows' milk formula should still be used. From about one year, 'doorstep' whole pasteurised milk may be used. This need not be boiled, since boiling destroys much of the important vitamins. Hygiene remains essential, and feeding bottles should always be sterilised. Skimmed milk should not be used for children under five years, though in special cases semi-skimmed milk can be used after two years of age.

Changing from breast milk to cows' milk usually causes the stools to become firmer and more smelly. Solid foods also influence the nature of the stools. Thus cereals and banana may make the stools firmer, while most fruits tend to make them looser. Constipation should be treated by giving the baby more diluted fruit juice, or cooled boiled water and mashed or chopped vegetables, and not by giving extra sugar in the feeds. Aperients should not be necessary, and should never be given without medical supervision.

A baby may need more water during very hot weather. A breast fed baby, who may be unhappy about taking a bottle of extra fluids, can usually meet the demands of fluid loss by having more frequent breast feeds. To guard against dehydration, diluted baby fruit juices or cooled boiled water can be offered by spoon. Bottle fed babies should be offered extra drinks rather than extra milk feeds.

Bottles or 'feeders' should never be left with babies. This is dangerous, as they may choke, and it may contribute to the development of dental caries. The frequency and duration of contact between drinks and teeth is a prime factor in the development of dental decay, and drink times should always be kept as short as possible. This applies to so-called 'natural' baby fruit drinks as much as to other types.

Although there are wide variations, the first teeth often begin to erupt at about five months. By six to seven months, most babies can chew lumpy foods and attempt to drink from a cup. Some mothers find a plastic egg cup a good intermediate step, because the baby can see over the rim while drinking. Trainer cups can be helpful to the mother, because they cause less spillage. But the baby still has to learn at some time to drink from the edge of a cup, and should be encouraged every so often to take the cup without the sealed lid.

From about seven months, pieces of hard food such as crusts, peeled apple or carrot should be given to help teething, but the baby must never be left alone with these foods, since there is a risk of choking. At this age, babies may want to take an active part in feeding themselves. Participation at meals

TABLE 8.1 Suggested weaning schedule

EARLY A.M.	BREAKFAST	LUNCH	TEA	LATE P.M.
4 MONTHS				
Breast or bottle feed	1–2 teaspoons of Baby Rice mixed with milk from feed, plus breast or bottle feed.	Breast or bottle feed.	Breast or bottle feed.	Breast or bottle feed.
4½ MONTHS				
Breast or bottle feed.	2 teaspoons of Baby Rice mixed with milk from feed, plus breast or bottle feed.	1–2 teaspoons pureed or sieved vegetables, or pureed or sieved meat and vegetables, or the same amount from a ready-prepared baby food. Breast or bottle feed.	Breast or bottle feed.	Breast or bottle feed.
5 – 6 MONTHS				
Breast or bottle feed.	Baby Rice or cereal mixed with milk from feed, or pureed banana, or firm boiled egg yolk, plus breast or bottle feed.	Pureed or sieved meat or fish and vegetables, or ready-prepared baby food, followed by pureed fruit or a ready-prepared baby dessert. Drink of cooled boiled water or diluted baby fruit drink.	Mashed banana or pureed fruit, or a ready-prepared baby dessert. Breast or bottle feed.	Breast or bottle feed.
6 – 7 MONTHS				
Breast or bottle feed.	Cereal mixed with milk from feed. Boiled, poached or scrambled egg, or toast fingers spread with a little unsalted butter. Breast or bottle feed.	Finely minced meat or mashed filleted fish with mashed vegetables, or a ready-prepared baby meal. Mashed banana or mashed stewed fruit, or a milk pudding or ready-prepared baby dessert. Drink of cooled boiled water or diluted baby fruit drink.	Lightly buttered toast with a cheese or savoury spread, or sandwiches with a cheese or savoury spread filling. Breast or bottle feed.	
7 – 8 MONTHS				
Breast or bottle feed.	Cereal, fish or an egg. Lightly buttered toast. Milk.	Minced meat, liver, chicken or mashed fish with mashed vegetables, or ready-prepared baby food. Milk pudding or stewed or mashed fruit, or ready-prepared baby dessert. Drink of cooled, boiled water or diluted baby fruit drink.	Toast or sandwiches with cheese or savoury spread filling, or mashed-up pasta with a cheesy sauce, or thick home-made soup, or ready-prepared baby food. Fruit or ready-prepared dessert, a sponge finger or a biscuit. Milk drink.	
9 – 12 MONTHS				
Breast or bottle feed.	Cereal and milk. Poached, scrambled or boiled egg, or a portion of poached or grilled filleted fish, and fingers of lightly buttered toast. Milk drink.	Well-chopped meat or liver, or fish or cheese with chopped or mashed vegetables, or ready-prepared baby meal. Milk pudding or fruit, or ready-prepared baby dessert. Drink of cooled boiled water or diluted baby fruit drink.	Fish, cheese or pasta suitably prepared, or savoury sandwiches, or toast with a savoury topping. Fruit. Milk drink.	

IMPORTANT Whichever way you serve eggs, they should be well cooked until firm all through, never soft or runny.

81

should be encouraged, and the baby should be given a spoon to 'help' the mother. This is usually a messy business, and a stiff pelican-type bib, with a curved bottom to catch spilt food, is a great help if the baby will wear it. A newspaper spread under the chair is also helpful. Parents who hinder this messy stage by preventing experimentation with foods may find that the child takes longer to become independent at mealtimes.

The suggested infant weaning schedule shown in Table 8.1 is a general guide to the kind of regimen which is appropriate, but it should be varied to suit the needs of individual children.

Overfeeding and the needlessly early introduction of solids should be discouraged. However, if the signs indicate that a baby is not satisfied after a feed, or if he is demanding more frequent feeds, then a small quantity of solid food may help to settle him, but should not be sufficient to cause excessive weight gain. No solids should ever be added to a bottle feed. Choking and, more rarely, inhalation pneumonia can result.

A body weight of approximately 14lb (6.5kg) is a good pointer to the commencement of solids, and should be considered in relation to the age of the baby. Not all babies at four months are ready, heavy or interested enough to commence solids safely. On the other hand, a baby of three months may weigh 14lb or more, and may be hungry and demanding, and the 'four month rule' should not then be too rigidly applied.

Vitamin supplements and trace elements

Vitamin supplements are recommended by the DHSS, and should be given to children from six months to five years. Early use of vitamin supplements (from one month) is still sometimes advised by professionals. Unless there is doubt about the vitamin intake of the breast feeding mother, however, the vitamin content of the breast milk, combined with the baby's own vitamin stores, should suffice until weaning is commenced. Bottle fed babies receive added vitamins in the milk formulas available in the U.K., and do not need further supplements until the milk formula is no longer given.

Families with special requirements

Not every family bases its main meal of the day on meat or fish and two vegetables. Different diets may be adopted for ethical, medical or religious reasons. For example, there are about a million vegetarians in the United Kingdom.[24]

The main difference between meat and vegetarian diets is the source of protein. Simply cutting out meat and fish, and substituting more eggs, cheese, baked beans and pizzas is not the complete answer. While in general, vegetarian and vegan diets are quite healthy if followed properly, pregnancy, lactation and rapid growth in childhood place extra demands on the body which must be met.

The term vegetarian covers a broad spectrum of eating, but all vegetarians exclude meat and fish. A **lacto-vegetarian** diet includes milk and milk products such as yogurt and cheese: an **ovo-lacto-vegetarian** diet also includes eggs. Vegans (strict vegetarians) eat no food of animal origin at all.

Weaning the vegetarian baby

In principle, weaning a baby onto a vegetarian diet is the same as weaning an omnivorous child. Small amounts of food should be offered, one type at a time, so that over a period of months a wide variety of food is accepted. If eggs and/or milk and milk products are included, nutritional requirements are easy to meet. With a stricter diet, there are problems that need to be considered.

Energy intake. Fruits, grains and vegetables are filling, but because of their fibre content, care needs to be taken that the child is receiving sufficient Calories.

Calcium and vitamin D. Food sources of these nutrients are limited, and so it is generally recommended that breast feeding should be continued for a longer time, or that a suitable soya based alternative, which includes added calcium and vitamin D, is used. (See list in Chaper 7.) However, not all soya based milks are suitable – one, Wysoy, contains fatty acids of animal origin – and unsupplemented plant based milks are not a suitable alternative to breast milk.

It is thought that strict vegans adapt to a low calcium intake. Certainly no cases of frank deficiency have been recorded. For other sources of calcium from plant foods, see Appendix.

A major source of vitamin D for vegan children is sunlight, but great caution needs to be exercised in recommending this, especially for very young or fair-skinned babies, since there is concern that over-exposure to sunlight may be a cause of the increasing incidence of skin cancers in adults and, in any event, babies burn and succumb to sunstroke easily. Some soya products contain added vitamin D, such as the plant sterol D_2, and so do vegan margarines such as 'Tomor'.

However, it is recommended that all vegan children under five years should receive supplements of vitamins A, D, C and B_{12}, and that vegan mothers should take supplements of vitamin D during pregnancy and while breast feeding.

Fibre intake. The fibre content of a vegan diet is higher than that of the average British diet, and may inhibit the absorption of important minerals like iron, calcium and zinc. It is therefore important that good sources of these are included each day.

Protein intake. Since protein is needed for growth, children have generally high requirements. About ten per cent of their energy intake should come from protein, and in the vegan diet this can be obtained from a variety of grains, nuts, pulse vegetables (especially soya beans), and potatoes. What is important is to balance the combination of different plant foods, so that the aminoacids of each complement the others. Pulses, for example, are low in methionine and cystine, but rich in lysine. Maize ('corn') is low in lysine, but has plenty of methionine and cystine. Many commercial weaning foods use this combination principle, for example by mixing soya flour with cereal. Pureed lentils and rice can make a suitable early weaning food.

Vitamin B_{12}. This is the vitamin most likely to be lacking in vegan diets. A deficiency leads to a macrocytic anaemia, which may be masked by a high intake of folic acid (not unusual with a vegan diet). In time, if deficiency signs are ignored, there is degeneration of the spinal cord.

Vitamin B_{12} is made exclusively by microorganisms, so it has been argued that it can be made in a healthy colon. However, there have been reports (cited[25]) of vitamin B_{12} deficiency in exclusively breast fed infants of vegan mothers. All plant foods are free of the vitamin, unless they have been contaminated by microorganisms or by insects. Exceptions to this general rule include *Spirulina*, an alga, some soy products such as miso and tempeh, some seaweeds, fortified yeast extracts (too salty for a young baby) and fortified plant milks. Breast feeding vegan mothers are recommended to take vitamin B_{12} supplements.

Iron. Although there are plenty of vegetable sources of iron, this iron is not so well absorbed as is iron from meat. The presence of vitamin C is important in a vegan or vegetarian diet, since it aids the absorption of iron from bread, pulses, nuts, and dark green leafy vegetables.

The vegan diet: summary

Many vegan children are breast fed well into their second year of life, and if the mother herself is well nourished, this is a good policy. However, deferring the introduction of other foods beyond the age of six months is not satisfactory. Assuming that a vegan baby has been weaned sensibly, and by the age of 9 to 12 months is eating the family meals, there is no reason why he should not be perfectly healthy. Although vegan children tend to be lighter and shorter than the average, there is no evidence to suggest that this is a health hazard, and indeed it may even be beneficial.

Very restricted diets are not recommended by the Vegan Society. A few recorded cases of frank infant malnutrition in this country (cited[26]) involved strict fruitarian and macrobiotic diets. In their extreme form, these diets are insufficient for children, since they contain too much bulk to allow the child to obtain adequate nourishment.

Fruitarian and macrobiotic diets

A fruitarian diet consists only of raw fruit, nuts and berries.

A macrobiotic diet may or may not be vegetarian, and is based on a classification of foods according to their 'Yin' and 'Yang' (positive and negative) properties. The classification includes factors such as colour, direction of growth (up or down), taste, season and weight. The originator is thought to be a Japanese, George Ohsawa, who has taken his philosophy from a number of Eastern religions, but particularly from Zen Buddhism.

In practice the diet is based largely on wholegrain cereals, of which it is said that 'they are the combination of both a fruit and a seed and contain a perfect balance of the nutrients needed for a healthy diet'.[3] Beans, soya products, vegetables, seaweeds and some 'wild' foods such as nettles, burdock and dandelion, can be added to provide variety and flavour.

Some fish, poultry, eggs and fruit may be eaten occasionally. Such a diet could be healthy for adults, but is probably too filling for young, rapidly growing children, who may not extract enough nutrients from macrobiotic foods.

Too early an introduction to a wholefood or macrobiotic diet, even of the best kind, is risky for the health of the growing child, as these diets can be nutritionally inadequate. Net protein utilisation is low, and such children are at risk from vitamin and mineral deficiencies. Cases of malnutrition in children following such diets have been reported (cited[27]).

Vegetarian sources of various nutrients

Important note: Babies can easily choke on nuts or some seeds, even if they seem finely chopped. Where nuts or seeds are listed below, it should be understood that they must be very finely ground or made into a smooth paste.

Where **yeast extracts** are listed, it should be remembered that they may be too salty for children under six months. Even after that age, they should be used in *very small* quantities only.

Note that not all soya based milks are suitable for vegans, as some contain fatty acids of animal origin. Unsupplemented plant based milks are not suitable for infants as an alternative to breast milk.

Concentrated energy (high Calorie foods). Nuts, nut butters and creams. Margarines and oils. Milk substitutes. Sunflower or sesame seeds, milled or made into spreads. Avocado pear.

Protein combinations. Baked beans and bread or toast. Rice and lentils. Smooth peanut butter and bread or toast. Nut roast (nuts and breadcrumbs). Soya and cereals. Seeds and cereals, such as sesame seed spread (tahini) on bread. Oatmeal and nuts, e.g. muesli.

Zinc. Nuts – especially Brazils, almonds, peanuts, hazelnuts and walnuts. Cereals – wheat, oats and rye.

Iron. Pulses, especially soya. Soya flour. Nuts. Sesame and pumpkin seeds. Cereals, e.g. millet, wheat, oats, bread, oatmeal, muesli. Wheat germ. Yeast extracts. Cocoa. Molasses and black treacle. Dark green leafy vegetables – broccoli, kale, watercress, parsley, spinach. Dried fruits. Fortified infant foods.

Vitamin C. Citrus fruits and their juices. Berry fruits: blackcurrants, raspberries, strawberries, loganberries. Salad vegetables: red and green peppers, watercress, bean sprouts, mustard and cress, tomatoes, radish, sorrell. Green leafy vegetables (quickly cooked). Potatoes, especially new potatoes. Parsley. Lychees, mangoes. Kiwi fruit.

Vitamin B group. Wholegrain cereals, e.g. wholemeal bread. Fortified breakfast cereals. Fortified infant foods. Yeast extracts. Wheat germ. Fresh vegetables: greens and potatoes.

Vitamin B_{12}. Fortified yeast extracts, e.g. 'Barmene', 'Tastex'. Fortified soya milks. Fortified breakfast cereals. Fortified textured vegetable protein (TVP). Fortified infant foods.

Calcium. Nuts, especially almonds. Green leafy vegetables, especially watercress and spinach. 'Hard' water. Sesame seeds and spreads (tahini). Cereals such as millet. Fortified bread. Fortified plant based milks. Baking powder. Molasses and black treacle (these are sugar products and should be used sensibly). Pulses.

Vitamin D. Fortified margarines. Fortified infant foods. Some breakfast cereals. Some malted milk drinks.

Cooking beans

It is essential that beans are pre-soaked and boiled for at least ten minutes in order to destroy natural toxins. A slow cooker should not be used, but a pressure cooker is ideal. The problem of flatulence created by eating beans is minimised if they are soaked in cold water first, and this water is discarded before cooking. Salt (for adults only) and other seasonings should be added after cooking, because the addition of salt while cooking makes the skins tough.

References

1. DHSS, 1988. Present Day Practice in Infant Feeding: Third Report. Report on Health and Social Subjects 32. HMSO
2. Harker P, Clark R, Thorogood M and Mann J, 1979. Infant Feeding Confusion. Nursing Times, Community Outlook, (2), 17-18
3. Wilkinson P W and Davies D P, 1978. When and Why are Babies Weaned? British Medical Journal, 1, 1682–1683
4. Barrie H, 1978. Letter: British Medical Journal, 2, 633
5. Poskitt E M E and Cole T J, 1978. Nature, Nurture and Childhood Overweight. British Medical Journal, 1, 603-605
6. Agras W S, Karaemer H C, Berkowitz R I et al, 1987. Does a Vigorous Feeding Style Influence Early Development of Obesity? The Journal of Pediatrics, **110**, (5), 799–804
7. Decreased Energy Expenditure as a Cause of Obesity in Infants, 1988. Nutrition Reviews, **46** (7) (July), 255–257
8. Tanner J M, Whitehouse T H and Tahaishi M, 1966. Standards from Birth to Maturity for Height, Weight and Weight Velocity in British Children. Archives of Disease in Childhood, **41**, 454
9. Peckham C S, Stark O, Simonite V and Wolff O H, 1983. Prevalence of Obesity in British Children born in 1946 and 1958. British Medical Journal, **286**, 1237–42
10. DHSS, 1980. Present Day Practice in Infant Feeding. Report on Health and Social Subjects, 20. HMSO
11. Aukett M A, Parks Y A, Scott P H and Wharton B A, 1986. Treatment with Iron Increases Weight Gain and Psychomotor Development. Archives of Disease in Childhood, **61**, 849–857
12. Grindulis H, Scott P H, Belton N R and Wharton B A, 1986. Combined Deficiency of Iron and Vitamin D in Asian Toddlers. Archives of Disease in Childhood, **61**, 843–848
13. Pollitt E, Saco-Pollitt C, Leibel R and Viteri F, 1986. Iron Deficiency and Behavioural Development in Infants and Pre-School Children. American Journal of Clinical Nutrition, **43**, 555–565
14. Tunnessen W W and Oski F, 1987. Consequences of Starting Whole Cow Milk at 6 Months of Age. Journal of Pediatrics, **111**, (6), 813–816
15. Fashakin J B and Oladimeji S, 1986. Effect of Ascorbic Acid on the Availability of Iron in Weaning Foods. Annals of Nutrition and Metabolism, **30**, 324–330
16. DHSS, 1984. Diet and Cardiovascular Disease. Report on Health and Social Subjects 28. HMSO
17. Ashbrook S and Doyle M. Infants' Acceptance of Strong- and Mild-Flavoured Vegetables. Journal of Nutrition Education, 17, (1), 5–6
18. Block S A, 1987. Prospective Appraisal of Complaints of Adverse Reactions to Foods in Children During the First 3 Years of Life. Pediatrics, **79**, 683–688
19. David T J, 1988. Food Additives. Archives of Disease in Childhood, **63**, 582–583

20. Coveney J, 1985. Is Breast Milk the Best Food for All Infants? Human Nutrition: Applied Nutrition, **39A**, (3), 179–188
21. Manual of Dietetic Practice (ed Thomas), 1988. British Dietetic Association. Blackwell Scientific Publications
22. National Advisory Committee on Nutrition Education, 1983. Proposals for Nutritional Guidelines for Health Education in Britain. Health Education Council.
22a. Wharton B A, 1987. Nutrition in the 1980's. In: Nutrition and Health, 5, 211–220
23. Fairweather-Tait S J, 1986. Iron Availability: the implications of short-term regulation. Nutrition Bulletin 48. British Nutrition Foundation, 11, (3), 174–180
24. Sanders T A B, 1988. Vegetarian and Macrobiotic Diets. Midwife, Health Visitor and Community Nurse, **24**, (5), 154–155
25. Langley C and Langley G, 1987. Infant Nutrition. The Vegan, New Series, **3**, (3), 7 and 13
26. Sams C, 1972. About Macrobiotics – the Way of Eating. Publ. Thorsons
27. Francis D, 1986. Nutrition for Children. Publ. Blackwell Scientific Publications

Further reading

Sarah Brown's Vegetarian Cookbook, 1987. Publ. Dorling Kindersley

Louise Templeton, 1985. The Right Food for Your Kids. Publ. Century

Publications from The Vegetarian Society, 53 Marloes Road, London W8, The Vegan Society Ltd., 33-35 George Street, Oxford OX1 2AY, and The Vegan Shop, 86 Tilehurst Road, Reading, Berks. RG3 2LU

Sylvia Hull, 1976. Cooking for a Baby. A Mother and Baby Publication. Publ. The Illustrated Publications Co. Ltd.

Sally Parsonage and June Clark, 1981. Infant Feeding and Family Nutrition. HM & M Publishers

Edward and Wendy Esko, 1984. Macrobiotic Cooking for Everyone. Publ. Japan Publications Inc.

Keith Michell's Practically Macrobiotic Cookbook, 1987. Publ. Thorsons

CHAPTER 9

Low birth weight and dysmature infants and twins

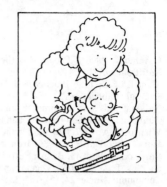

Babies having a birth weight of less than 2500g (5½ lb) and a gestation of less than 37 weeks are considered low birth weight (LBW). Those under 1500g with a gestational age of less than 33 weeks are classed as very low birth weight (VLBW) and especially high risk. Where modern special care baby units are available the survival rate is steadily improving, and most low birth weight babies develop normally.

Low birth weight infants (short gestation)

The weight, length and development at birth correspond to the period of gestation. Thus the infant's head is disproportionately large and the respiratory, heat regulatory, neuromuscular and digestive systems are immature.

Intensive care is invariably essential owing to the high risks related to immaturity of organ function. These include asphyxia, respiratory distress syndrome, brain damage, immature kidney function and acute susceptibility to temperature changes. Survival rates have generally shown an improvement since 1965, but mortality varies according to the geographical area, medical services available, social class of population, and the frequency of very low birth weight infants in a particular area. Chances of survival definitely improve with a higher gestational age.

The following problems arise as a result of the immature physiology of short gestation infants:

1 Sucking and swallowing reflexes are poorly developed, so there is a tendency to regurgitate the stomach contents.

2 The baby cannot adjust to changes in the environmental temperature, and therefore quickly becomes overheated or chilled. Incubator care is frequently required.

3 There is a marked susceptibility to infection.

4 Poor liver function gives rise to jaundice.

5 Kidney function is feeble and the acid-base balance is readily disturbed. Water retention may occur.

6 The lungs are immature, breathing is irregular, and there is a likelihood of developing idiopathic respiratory distress syndrome.

7 Enzyme systems are poorly developed so that digestion is easily upset by large feeds.

The surviving premature infant is at greater risk from disabilities such as delay in development, visual, hearing and speech impairments, hydrocephalus and cerebral palsy. Most handicaps are diagnosed early, but some prove to be more difficult, such as learning disorders and abnormal behaviour. The lower the birth weight the greater the chance of handicap.

Management

An infant born prematurely at home should be transferred immediately to the nearest special care baby unit, unless the birth weight is more than 2000g (4lb 7oz) and the baby is obviously lively. Larger infants should be moved to hospital if the home circumstances are poor or if complications, such as hypothermia, develop. The baby should always be moved in a portable incubator.[1]

The decision as to how and when to start feeding LBW infants is a controversial one. Most authorities agree that the first feed should be given when the infant is between 12 and 24 hours old. Babies weighing 1500g (3lb 5oz) or more may be allowed to suck from a bottle. Smaller infants, or those who are ill, require feeding by tube. Tube feeding should be slowly replaced with a bottle when the baby shows signs of sucking. Breast feeding is rarely initially successful with infants weighing less than 2000g (4lb 7oz) but can be tried under close supervision with all necessary safeguards for the baby. More usually the baby will be fed the mother's undiluted breast milk within a few hours of birth, the quantity being increased daily.[2] A supply of breast milk may be maintained by manual expression until the infant is strong enough to be fed at the breast.

The initial feed should be boiled water or 10% glucose water, and if the water is retained, milk used for subsequent feeds. Most paediatricians agree that breast milk is particularly suitable for LBW infants, but many now prefer the specially formulated low soluble milks for the very low birth weight baby.

Most premature infants require 540 kJ (130 kcal) per kilogram body weight per day (200ml milk per kilogram of body weight per day) but the aim must be to give as much milk as the infant will tolerate without regurgitation, and the optimum quantity of feed will vary with individual infants.

Calculating feeds for the premature infant

The growth rate of the low birth weight baby is greater than that of the mature baby, and the amount of feed usually starts at 60ml/kg body weight per day in the first 24 hours, increasing by 30ml/kg body weight per day until 150ml/kg is reached on the fifth day.

Very small babies (under 1200g) may need 200ml/kg or more. Larger babies gain weight on smaller volumes, but on occasions may need over 200ml/kg body weight. The first feed should be boiled water, and feeding should commence within four hours of birth to prevent damage to the developing brain by jaundice, dehydration and hypoglycaemia.

Vitamin supplements

It is recommended that vitamins are started when the infant is between one and two weeks old. Vitamin D (1000 units daily), vitamins A and C, and possibly vitamin B are required. For small babies, Abidec (3 drops twice daily) is commenced at four weeks old.

Iron is not normally given until four weeks of age, as it is not well tolerated. Sytron (10 drops daily) is then prescribed. Later a folic acid supplement (50μg daily) may be required.

Dysmature infants (light-for-dates)

Any infant whose birth weight is below the tenth centile for gestational age is classified as dysmature.

These are infants who are poorly nourished *in utero* and are often starving when born. Dysmature infants have a mature physiology and therefore they are easier to feed than short gestation infants of similar weight.

The management of the dysmature infant is generally the same as that for the short gestation infant. However, there is one important difference. The dysmature infant should be given the first feed within two hours of birth, and not later than four hours after birth. Early feeding is essential if hypoglycaemia is to be avoided.

The first feed should consist of glucose water, and for subsequent feeds either expressed breast milk or a suitable formula milk is usually recommended.

A three-hourly schedule may be necessary, and the quantity of milk given per feed should be sufficient to satisfy the infant's demand. This may be considerably more than the volume consumed by a premature infant of similar weight.

Initially a large milk intake as high as 200ml/kg per day will be taken, but by the second or third week the extreme hunger subsides and the quantities required will approach the normal intake of 150ml/kg per day.

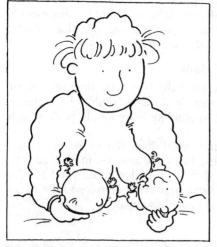

Breast feeding twins

Feeding twins

Twins may be of average birth weight but are often smaller. The management of twins whose birth weight is under 2500g (5lb 7oz), and who are premature or dysmature, is the same as that of any low birth weight baby and has been discussed above.

Simultaneous breast feeding is the most satisfactory, and the best position is to have the heads of the babies forward with their legs behind the mother. The mother supports their heads with her hands, aided by a pillow. However, twins are individuals and may be better suited by individual feeding as required, if the mother can cope with the demand on her time. Usually some compromise is needed. Domestic help for the mother is most desirable, especially in the early weeks, and she needs adequate rest and a good diet.

References

1. Forfar J O et al, 1973. The Newborn. In: Textbook of Paediatrics, eds. Forfar J O and Arneil G C. Publ. Churchill Livingstone, Edinburgh
2. Davies D P, 1978. The First Feed of Low Birth-Weight Infants. Archives of Disease in Childhood, 53, 187

See also: Mayes Midwifery: Textbook for Midwives, revised Sweet B R, 1982

CHAPTER 10

Some problems
associated with feeding

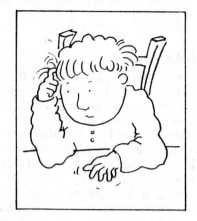

Allergy to milk

Allergy to human milk is extremely rare but not unknown.[1,2] Allergy to cows' milk is rare. The main symptoms include rhinitis (runny nose), eczema, abdominal pain, vomiting, diarrhoea and wheezing. Infantile allergy is a temporary problem and most children grow out of it by the age of 2 to 3 years.

Management of cows' milk allergy involves replacement of foods containing cows' milk or cows' milk products in the infant's diet with one of the specialised alternative infant formulae, which include the soya formulae Cow & Gate Formula 'S', Pro-Sobee, Isomil, Ostersoy and Wysoy. Parents must be advised to ask for them by name because they are the only soya formula foods suitable for infant feeding, the other soya products available in grocers and supermarkets being nutritionally inadequate for feeding babies. These five named brands can be obtained on prescription in the United Kingdom if a diagnosis of cows' milk allergy has been established.

Despite popular acclaim, goats' milk has no special value in the management of cows' milk allergy. The high protein and mineral content of goats' milk means that it is unsuitable for babies under the age of six months.

Severe cases of cows' milk allergy, involving damage to the absorptive surface of the intestine, should be managed with a formula in which the protein has been hydrolysed (pre-digested). Pregestimil (Mead Johnson) is the chosen product for infants aged less than six months, whereas Nutramigen (Mead Johnson) is suitable for older babies and children. Both Pregestimil and Nutramigen should be used only on the advice of a doctor or dietitian.

Cows' milk allergy is fully discussed in *Food Allergy* (publ. Edsall, 1980).

Cleft palate

One baby in every 700 born in the UK is affected by cleft lip and/or cleft palate. Although breast feeding may be difficult, it is often not impossible for the mother who perseveres. A great advance has been made in bottle feeding by the Haberman Feeder, which is now regarded as the best method of feeding these babies.[3] The feeder is activated by tongue pressure rather than suction, and it delivers feed in quantities controlled by the baby. If the baby needs help, gentle finger pressure on the reservoir delivers a small quantity of feed at a time. Simple rotation of the teat in the mouth will reduce or stop the flow altogether, enabling a baby to get used to the feel of the teat before feeding begins. Its unique design helps to reduce wind and to cut oral feeding

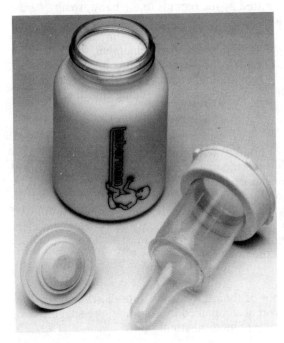

The Haberman Feeder

time by up to 80 per cent. The feeder is also indicated in cases of prematurity, heart conditions, cerebral palsy, Downs syndrome and Pierre Robin syndrome.

Other feeding methods for babies with cleft palate include a special hooded teat, a pipette with catheter, or a spoon.

Coeliac disease

This is a fairly rare condition, also known as gluten enteropathy, in which the lining of the small intestine is damaged by gluten, the cereal protein found in wheat, rye, barley and oats. When one of these cereals is given, the baby may vomit, develop pale, bulky motions, suffer from anaemia and vitamin deficiencies, and go off his food. In addition the stomach may swell and there will be a loss in weight gain. The treatment is to remove all gluten from the diet. The child will then recover, but the gluten-free diet may have to be followed throughout life.

Colic

This term is used to describe symptoms which indicate acute abdominal pain. The baby draws up the legs, screams and cries, and cannot be comforted. These symptoms occur fairly commonly in the first three months of life.

There is no completely satisfactory hypothesis as to why this condition occurs but hunger is the commonest cause, while food allergy, air swallowing, and tension and anxiety transmitted by the parents to the baby are among the factors which should be considered.

A doctor may prescribe a relaxant drug (dicyclomine dihydrochloride)[4] to relieve the baby's discomfort. It is important to remember that a crying, irritable baby who cannot be comforted is extremely tiring and exasperating, and may be in danger of abuse from a fraught parent. It is therefore necessary to give the parents counselling support as well as seeing that the baby has treatment.

Constipation

(a) Absence of stools for 24 hours is not significant. (b) In cases of excessive dryness of stools due to underfeeding or excessive sweating, additional fluid should be given. (c) Spasm of the anal sphincter may be relieved by gentle dilatation by a trained person using the (lubricated) finger tip. (d) In spite of the media publicity given to fibre in the diet, parents should be cautioned about its over-use for children under one year of age. Sufficient fluids should be given, including water. Aperients must be avoided. Toilet training should start only after the first year.

Diarrhoea

(a) Small, loose stools do not of themselves constitute diarrhoea. (b) Frequent watery stools, especially if accompanied by vomiting, are suggestive of gastroenteritis which calls for urgent medical attention.

Dehydration

Dehydration is most likely to occur in the first six months after birth if a baby either has had an inadequate fluid intake, or has lost an excessive volume of fluid, although it can occur in older babies. The symptoms and signs are: (a) restlessness; (b) dry skin and mucous membranes; (c) temperature rise as high as 40 deg. C (104 deg. F); (d) tongue papillae enlarged and red; and (e) scanty urine. If the condition does not subside when extra fluids are given, medical attention is urgently required.

Drugs

The possibility that the mother is taking drugs, either on prescription or otherwise, which are harmful to the baby's well-being, should not be overlooked.

Eczema (see Skin eruptions)

Fat intolerance (mild)

Diarrhoea is present, resulting in soreness around the anus, which causes crying or screaming on defaecation. Medical attention is required.

Fat intolerance (severe)

Stools are large, pale, loose and offensive, resembling coeliac disease. Medical attention is required.

94

Nasal obstruction

Excessive humidity will cause excessive nasal secretion and will inhibit feeding. Medical advice should be sought if the secretion becomes thick or purulent. There is a risk of bronchitis.

Overfeeding

The baby regurgitates large amounts of milk and is unhappy between feeds, crying and flexing the hips. Several large stools are passed causing sore buttocks. This is entirely a question of management and the mother should be helped accordingly.

Possetting and regurgitation of food

The cause may be air swallowing or too much food. Prevention is possible by avoiding movement and manipulation after feeds. Alternatively the cause may be a temporary laxity of the cardia of the stomach (oesophageal reflux).

Protein intolerance (mild)

This condition is uncommon and does not occur in breast fed babies. The symptoms are vomiting, crying, restlessness, failure to gain weight, and large stringy pale curds in the vomit and stools. Specially prepared milks are usually prescribed.

Skin eruptions

Rashes and eruptions of the skin are common and often transient in babies. They are often inaccurately labelled eczema. This can cause unnecessary anxiety to parents, who should be reassured that if indeed their baby has eczema, it is not catching, will not leave scars on the skin, and usually clears up by the age of two or three years.

Eczema (from the Greek 'I boil') appears on the forehead and cheeks as dry red patches. The flexures of the elbows and behind the knees and ears are other common sites. Weeping occurs in more severe cases followed by crust formation. Itching is a feature. The causes are not fully understood, but eczema appears to be an allergic condition and may be aggravated by wool, detergents, and washing the skin with soap and water. If sensitivity to cows' milk protein is a factor, soya-based milk or hydrolysed protein milk is sometimes substituted. The doctor may prescribe cortisone cream and emulsifying ointments.

Thrush

Infection due to *Candida albicans*. Not only will this interfere with feeding, but the infection can spread throughout the gastro-intestinal tract. Medical treatment may be necessary and the source of infection will require investigation. The doctor may prescribe an oral suspension drug to be dropped into the baby's mouth three times daily.

Underfeeding

The baby is a ravenous feeder, waking well before a feed is due. Air swallowing causes flatulence, vomiting and colic. The stools are small in number and quantity, and dark green. The weight gain is poor. This can almost always be solved by helping the mother to manage the feeding properly.

Alternatively, the baby may appear contented and sleep most of the time, the poor weight gain being the only sign of underfeeding.[5]

Vomiting

This is a sign calling for examination to exclude: (a) hypertrophic pyloric stenosis; (b) atresia of the oesophagus; (c) congenital causes of obstruction lower in the intestinal tract; (d) meconium ileus, which is due to the loss of the lubricating action of the meconium when the latter has an abnormal viscosity and cannot pass into the large intestine; (e) imperforate anus; (f) hiatus hernia; (g) infectious illnesses, e.g. gastroenteritis; (h) urinary tract infection.

References

1. Gerrard J W, 1979. Allergy in Breast Fed Babies to Ingredients in Breast Milk. Annals of Allergy, 42, 269–78
2. Wergeland H, 1948. Three Fatal Cases of Probable Familial Allergy to Human Milk. Acta Paediatrica Scandanavica, 35, 321–334
3. Campbell A N and Trenouth M J, 1987. New Feeder for Infants with Cleft Palate. Archives of Disease in Childhood, 62, 1292
4. McKeith R and Wood C, 1977. Infant Feeding and Feeding Difficulties. 5th edn. Publ. Churchill Livingstone, Edinburgh
5. Illingworth R S, 1983. The Normal Child. Publ. Churchill Livingstone, Edinburgh

Appendix

Good sources of vitamin A

Liver – ox, pigs, calves, lamb and chicken;
Fatty fish – mackerel, herring, sardines, salmon;
Vegetables – carrots, tomatoes, most dark green leafy vegetables such as watercress, spinach, kale etc.;
Fruit – apricots, pineapple, peach, nectarine;
Butter, margarine, cheese, full fat milk and cream.

In vegetables and fruits, the vitamin A is in the form of the 'precursor', carotene. It is converted to vitamin A in the body.

Other sources of vitamin A include: cod and halibut liver oils, malt with cod liver oil, Welfare vitamin drops and tablets, multivitamin tablets.

Good sources of vitamin D

Sunlight – converts 7-dehydrocholesterol in the skin to cholecalciferol, which undergoes subsequent changes in the liver and in the kidneys to form the active substance, 1,25 di-hydroxycholecalciferol. Vitamin D acts more like a hormone than a vitamin, but cholecalciferol (vitamin D_3) can be found in a few foods:

Cod liver oil, Halibut oil, Welfare vitamin drops and tablets;

Fatty fish – eels, herrings, kippers, mackerel, salmon, brislings and sardines;

Malt with cod liver oil, margarine which is fortified with vitamin D, egg yolks, dried and evaporated milks which are fortified, some brands of natural yogurt, some brands of malted milk drinks.

Butter, liver, milk and cheese contain only a little vitamin D.

Good sources of vitamin C

Blackcurrants, strawberries, rosehip syrup, blackcurrant syrups, kiwi fruit, watercress, mustard and cress, green peppers, mangetout, beansprouts, broccoli, brussels sprouts, cabbage, cauliflower, kale, parsley, spinach, turnip tops.

Citrus fruits (oranges, lemons, tangerines, grapefruit), redcurrants, raspberries, gooseberries, potatoes (especially new), broad beans, asparagus.

Blackberries, limes, melon, fresh pineapple, runner beans, peas (fresh or frozen), tomatoes, liver, roe.

Welfare vitamin drops and tablets.

Vegetables that are to be cooked need to be cooked quickly, and not kept warm before eating, so that maximum vitamin C is retained.

Dried fruits and vegetables, processed peas, and jams are not good sources of vitamin C.

Good sources of vitamin B_1 (thiamin)

Yeast and yeast extracts, wholemeal bread and cereals, breakfast cereals that are fortified, wheatgerm, oatmeal, pork, peas and potatoes, most red meats, milk, peanuts.

Large amounts of thiamin may be lost in processing and cooking.

Good sources of vitamin B_2 (riboflavin)

Yeast and yeast extracts, wholemeal breads and cereals, wheat bran and germ, fresh pulse vegetables (peas and beans), meat (especially kidney, liver, heart etc.), fish, eggs, cheese, milk, natural yogurts, oatmeal, nuts, green vegetables, beer.

Riboflavin is destroyed by alkaline conditions and by exposure to ultraviolet light.

Good sources of nicotinic acid (niacin)

Meats (all kinds), fish (all kinds), wholemeal breads and cereals, peas and beans, coffee.

Milk and eggs are good sources of the amino acid tryptophan, which is converted to nicotinic acid in the body.

Good sources of vitamin B_6 (pyridoxine)

Meats (especially liver and kidney), egg yolk, peas and beans, wholegrain breads and cereals, fresh fish, some fresh fruits (especially bananas and avocado pears), some dried fruits.

Most vegetables contain some vitamin B_6. Several drugs antagonise the action of vitamin B_6, notably the oral contraceptive pill, isoniazid, hydralazine and penicillamine. So do alcohol and cigarette smoking.

Good sources of folic acid (folate, folacin)

Dark green leafy vegetables such as spinach, broccoli, kale, spring greens, Savoy cabbage etc.

Liver and kidney, nuts, wholemeal breads and cereals.

Milk and dairy products supply some.

Vegetables should be cooked quickly, and in as little water as possible, in order to retain the maximum amount of folic acid.

Good sources of vitamin B_{12} (cyanocobalamin)

All foods of animal origin supply vitamin B_{12}. The richest sources include: liver, heart, kidney (all meats), fatty fish, shellfish and white fish, eggs, milk and cheese.

Some breakfast cereals and malted milk drinks have added vitamin B_{12}. So do some yeast extracts, especially those manufactured for strict vegetarians (vegans). Some seaweeds and algae contain vitamin B_{12} and some soya protein products have it added.

A list of foods specially prepared for vegans is obtainable from the Vegan Society.

Other B-group vitamins such as biotin, pantothenic acid, choline and carnitine are found in a very wide variety of foods, and it is not considered necessary to list the sources here.

Good sources of zinc

Meat (all kinds), milk, natural yogurt, cheese, eggs, fish.

Wholemeal grains, peas, beans, nuts and a variety of vegetables also contain zinc, but it is not absorbed so well by the body. It is possible that vegans, who eat no animal foods at all, may adapt over a period of time to absorbing zinc better from grains, pulses and vegetables.

Good sources of iron

Red meats such as beef and lamb; corned beef;
Liver, heart, kidney, liver sausage and pates;
Black sausage;
Fatty fish – sardines, herrings, sprats, pilchards, mackerel;
Whitebait, mussels, winkles;
Soya beans.

There is a little iron in white meats such as chicken, and in white fish, which is well absorbed.

The following foods contain iron, but absorption is poor: wholegrain cereals, peas, beans and other pulses, cocoa, curry powder, eggs, nuts, some green vegetables such as spinach and watercress.

Good sources of calcium

Milks (all kinds), cheeses (all kinds except cream cheeses), natural yogurt;

Bread made from white, brown and wheatgerm flours (not wholemeal);

Tinned fish, e.g. sardines, tinned salmon etc., which contain soft bones that are safe to eat;

Hard water;

Some nuts and seeds, such as almonds and sesame seeds, but absorption of calcium from these may be poor, due to the presence of phytic acid;

Dark green vegetables, such as spinach, watercress and beetroot tops contain calcium, but the presence of oxalic acid may prevent good absorption.

Useful reading

The Everyman Companion to Food and Nutrition, 1987. Sheila Bingham. Publ. J M Dent & Sons

Index